Editoria

GW00976012

Protocol for Adminis
via Enteral Fe

1st edition, February 2000   ... namS.

2nd edition, April 2002   - Jen Smyth, MRPharmS.

3rd edition (internal only), May 2003   - Jen Smyth, MRPharmS.

4th edition, January 2004   - Jen Smyth, MRPharmS.

The NEWT Guidelines
for administration of medication to patients
with enteral feeding tubes or swallowing difficulties

1st edition, January 2006   - Jen Smyth, MRPharmS.

The information in this book is intended as a guide to administration of medication to patients with swallowing problems. Such administration is usually outside the product licence.

North East Wales NHS Trust does not authorise or take responsibility for any such administration, which should only be done with prescriber agreement, and a full understanding of the legal implications of medication administration outside the product licence.

Published by North East Wales NHS Trust,
Pharmacy Department, Wrexham Maelor Hospital,
Wrexham, North Wales, LL13 7TD.
ISBN 0-9552515-0-8
ISBN 978-0-9552515-0-4

Every reasonable attempt has been made to ensure
that the information in this guide is accurate and up to date
at the time of printing.

Acknowledgments

This guide is a compilation of theoretical, practical, and anecdotal information from a variety of sources. Many thanks to everyone who has contributed, particularly those people who have provided practical information to supplement previously theoretical guides. I would particularly like to mention the following sources, which have made significant contributions to this and previous editions.

Whipps Cross Hospital's Tube Feeding Drug Administration Guide.[40]

Derriford Hospital Pharmacy enteral feeding guide.[41]

Queen Victoria Hospital's Drug Adminstration via Enteral Feeding Tubes guide, March 2001.[94]

Southern General Hospital, South Glasgow University Hospitals NHS Trust's A to Z guide to administration of drugs via nasogastric/PEG tube. Updated June 2001.[95]

County Durham and Darlington Acute Hospitals NHS Trust's Guidelines for the administration of Drugs through Enteral Feeding Tubes, 2nd edition. July 2003.[104]

Stockport NHS Trust's Drugs via Enteral Feeding Tubes Guide (draft).[105]

Gloucestershire Hospitals NHS Foundation Trust's Guide to administration of medicines to patients with swallowing difficulties or feeding tubes (NG/PEG). Nov. 2004.[132]

Poole Hospital NHS Trust Pharmacy's Drug Administration Guidelines. July 2002.[133]

Calderdale and Huddersfield NHS Trust's Medication and Enteral Feeding. Feb. 2004.[135]

Mid Essex Hospitals Services NHS Trust's The Administration of medication via a Percutaneous Endoscopic Gastrostomy (PEG) tube. March 2002.[138]

I am also very grateful for the work on tablet dispersal carried out for this edition by Peter Bradshawe, Hannah Collins, and Brian Collins; the audit work undertaken by Elizabeth Alexander; the support of the North East Wales NHS Trust Nutritional Support Team and members of the Dietetics Department; and the help of the staff of Wrexham Maelor Hospital Pharmacy Department with compiling this document.

Jen Smyth, Editor.

New features in this edition

Welcome to the 1st edition of 'The NEWT Guidelines for administration of medication to patients with enteral feeding tubes or swallowing difficulties.' (previously the 'Protocol for Administration of Medication via Enteral Feeding Tubes.')

This book is the result of continued work by the staff of the Pharmacy Department of Wrexham Maelor Hospital, North East Wales NHS Trust, and the suggestions of the many users of the guidelines. It conforms to the same general layout as previous editions, but has some changes which should make it easier to use.

New monographs
This edition contains more than a hundred new drug monographs.

Patients with swallowing difficulties
This edition contains clearer sections containing specific advice for patients with swallowing difficulties, separate from the sections on enteral feeding tubes, and some general guidance on the problems associated with administering medicines to patients with swallowing difficulties.

Feed guidance
This edition contains separate sections indicating guidance for enteral feeding in association with medicines administration when the administration of medicines may require adjustment of the feed.

Drug names
All drugs are listed by their recommended names following the changes from British Approved Names (BAN) to Recommended International Non-proprietary Names (RINN).

Tablet dispersal
This edition includes the results of tablet dispersal testing work carried out in-house, providing more specific information regarding the length of time required for tablet dispersal.

Monograph Layout

Each drug monograph should be read in conjunction with the notes on administration (section 3). The monographs are laid out as follows:-

Presentation
The available formulation presentations for each drug are listed at the start of each monograph. The presence of the formulations here does not indicate that they are suitable for administration to patients with enteral feeding tubes or swallowing difficulties, but is merely a guide to what is available.

Some formulations may be unlicensed 'specials' available only at some centres, and sometimes having to be ordered in on a named patient basis.

Administration – enteral tubes / swallowing difficulties
Some monographs have a combined administration section, when the guidance for patients with enteral feeding tubes can equally be applied to patients with swallowing difficulties.

Administration – enteral tubes
Some monographs have a separate section with specific guidance on how to administer via enteral feeding tubes.

Administration – swallowing difficulties
Some monographs have a separate section with specific guidance on how to administer to patients with swallowing difficulties.

Administration – NG / PEG tubes / swallowing difficulties
Where method of administration differs depending on whether the drug is delivered to the stomach or the jejunum, separate instructions are given.

Administration – NJ / PEJ / PEGJ tubes

Where method of administration differs depending on whether the drug is delivered to the stomach or the jejunum, separate instructions are given.

Clinical guidance

This important section lists any clinical problems which may commonly occur when medications are administered via enteral feeding tubes, or formulations are altered for patients with swallowing difficulties. It also indicates any monitoring which may be required (in addition, or more frequently, than would usually be the case).

Feed guidance

This section lists any known interactions with feeds (other than standard before / after food guidance which is commonly given with the listed medication), and any feeding breaks which may be advised when a patient is receiving the monograph medication.

Abbreviations

CR – controlled release

e/c – enteric-coated

mcg - micrograms

mg - milligrams

ml - millilitres

MR – modified release

NG - naso-gastric enteral feeding tube

NJ - naso-jejunal enteral feeding tube

PEG – percutaneous endoscopic gastrostomy enteral tube

PEGJ – percutaneous endoscopic gastro-jejunostomy enteral tube

PEJ – percutaneous jejunostomy enteral tube

Contents

1. Legal aspects of administering medication via enteral feeding tubes and altering formulations

Drug administration via enteral feeding tubes is almost always an unlicensed method of administration, therefore in all cases where a patient with an enteral feeding tube fitted requires oral medication, alternative (licensed) routes of administration should be sought. Medication designed and given via a licensed route of administration will produce a more predictable response than oral medicines given via an enteral feeding tube.[1]

The alteration of medication formulations (e.g. crushing tablets, opening capsules) to aid administration to patients with swallowing difficulties is also usually an unlicensed activity, with the same legal implications as medication administration via enteral feeding tubes.

When drug administration via enteral feeding tubes is necessary, the prescriber takes responsibility for the off-licence use of the drug concerned. According to the Medicines Act 1968, only a medical or dental practitioner can authorise the use of unlicensed medicines.[135] However the person administering the medication may still share some responsibility, even if they have written authority from the prescriber. Giving medicines via alternate routes (e.g. via enteral feeding tubes) or by alternate methods (e.g. crushing tablets) contrary to the directions of a prescriber is a breach of the Medicines Act 1968, and could result in a finding of professional misconduct.

Patient response to drugs administered via unlicensed routes can be unpredictable. Drugs may have a greater or lesser therapeutic effect than when given by the oral route. The onset and duration of effect may be affected. Side effects, particularly those involving the gastrointestinal system, are likely to be exacerbated. The side effects of drugs which have been given by an unlicensed route are also the responsibility of the prescriber.

If putting medication down an enteral feeding tube is unavoidable then it is sensible to keep drug therapy to a minimum. If problems do arise, please contact your Pharmacist who is in an ideal position to advise on the formulation, timing, and route of administration of drugs.

These guidelines are intended only as a guide to administration, and are **not** an authority for unlicensed administration of medication. The information contained in this guide is mostly anecdotal, as there is very little information on drug administration outside product licence.

Drugs should only be put down a feeding tube as a last resort because of the implications for drug therapy and nutritional status.

Consent

Every adult of sound mind who is able to give consent, must consent to administration of medication. Attempting to disguise medication ('covert administration') in such cases is a trespass against the person.[115] When a person is unable to give consent, such as when they are unconscious, or suffering from an impairment of mental functioning which leaves them unable to make informed decisions about their care, the law allows medicines to be given in the absence of consent, in the best interests of the patient. In England and Wales, relatives have no legal right to consent on behalf of incapable adults.[115]

2. Practical aspects of medication administration via enteral feeding tubes

2.1 Practical points

Tube types[137]

Nasogastric (NG) – inserted into the stomach via the nose.
Nasojejunal (NJ) – inserted into the jejunum via the nose. These tubes may also have a gastric port.
Percutaneous endoscopic gastrostomy (PEG) – inserted into the stomach via the abdominal wall.
Percutaneous endoscopic jejunostomy (PEJ) – inserted into the jejunum via the abdominal wall.
Percutaneous endoscopic gastro-jejunostomy (PEGJ) – inserted into the jejunum via the abdominal wall and through the stomach.

Nasogastric and naso-jejunal tubes are long fine bore tubes with a large surface area for potential drug absorption and may block easily due to their small bore. Percutaneous endoscopic gastrostomy, and jejunostomy tubes are short tubes with a wider bore.

When administering medicines via a tube that ends in the jejunum, sterile water should be used because the acid barrier in the stomach is by-passed. Drug absorption may be unpredictable if the tube extends beyond the drug's main site of absorption (e.g. cefalexin, ketoconazole).[137] There is a higher risk of diarrhoea with sorbitol-containing liquids and hypertonic solutions when administered directly into the jejunum as the buffering effect of the gastric contents is lost.[155]

Tube position

Tube tips can easily become dislodged by movement. Tube tip position should be tested using pH indicator paper, or according to local guidelines. Blue litmus paper is no longer considered to be appropriate for use, as it may not distinguish between bronichial and gastric placement.[118]

Tube tip position is most accurately checked by radiography, but in order to minimise exposure to radiation and to reduce handling of the patient, pH testing is the preferred method for most patients (excepting neonates). pH indicator strips should have 0.5 gradations and a range including 1-6. It is particularly important to be able to distinguish at the pH 5-6 range.[120]

Tube tip position should be checked: - [120]
- following initial insertion
- before administering each feed
- before giving medication
- at least once daily during continuous feeding
- following episodes of coughing, vomiting, or retching
- following evidence of tube displacement (e.g. more tube visible, loose tape)

pH testing results[120]

pH 5.5 or below – Commence feeding (there have been no reported cases of pulmonary aspirates below this figure).

pH above 6 – Do not feed. Wait 1 hour and try again (to allow feed to leave the stomach, and gastric acid levels to rise).

Patients on antacids, H_2 antagonists, or proton pump inhibitors may have gastric aspirates with pH of 6 or above. Seek advice and alternative methods of checking tube tip position in these patients if aspirate pH is high.[120]

General handling of enteral feeding tubes

Carers should wear gloves when handling enteral feeding tubes and preparing medicines for administration (e.g. when crushing tablets).

A 50ml oral, enteral, or catheter tipped syringe should be used for administration of medication.[112] Intravenous syringes should NOT be used due to the risk of accidental parenteral administration. The use of intravenous syringes has led to fatalities when medications for enteral use have been accidentally given intravenously.

Coloured enteral syringes are available in some centres. These may not be sterile, and may be re-used for the same patient. They should be clearly labelled with the patient details, and washed in hot soapy water immediately after each use, and allowed to dry in air. Immunocompromised patients and patients with enteral feeding tubes terminating in the jejunum may require the use of sterile equipment to reduce infection risk.

All equipment used for administering medicines must be cleaned in between each use to prevent cross-contamination of medicines. Particular care should be taken when handling drugs to which patients frequently suffer allergies, e.g. the penicillins.

Flushing enteral feeding tubes

Tube flushing should be done using a push-pause technique to create turbulence within the tube which helps to dislodge particles. Enteral feeding tubes should be flushed with 30ml of distilled water after the feed is stopped and before any medications are given, then with 10ml of distilled water between medications to prevent drug-drug interactions. When all the medications have been administered, flush the tube with at least 30ml of distilled water again before restarting the feed. This procedure reduces the risk of tube blockage and helps with the delivery of the drug to the stomach.[1] If the patient is fluid restricted, consult your Pharmacist or the Doctor.

Medications can react with the ions in tap water, therefore distilled water should be used for drug administration and enteral tube flushing unless otherwise directed. A separate bottle should be used for each patient, and discarded at the end of 24 hours.

Drug absorption via enteral feeding tubes

There are two main consequences for drug absorption via the stomach when an enteral feeding tube is in place.[1]

1. The delivery of drugs directly into the stomach bypasses the normal enteral route where saliva may assist degradation of the drug.

2. The residence time in the stomach is reduced. Absorption of drug will be impaired if prolonged contact with the acid environment of the stomach is required for drug dissolution. When an enteral tube terminating in the jejunum (NJ, PEJ, PEGJ) is used the acid environment of the stomach is bypassed altogether, which can result in only partial or no absorption of the drug.

Gastric motility and nasogastric suction

Gastric motility can inhibit absorption of medications administered via nasogastric or percutaneous gastrostomy tubes. If motility is believed to be a problem, referral to the local Nutrition team is advised.

Some drugs have been used to try and aid gastric motility through their pro-kinetic side effects. Metoclopramide (10mg three times a day) and erythromycin (250mg two or three times a day, preferably by the intravenous route) are the most commonly used.[90]

In patients with slow gastric emptying, it may be advisable to suspend nasogastric drainage / nasogastic suction following dosing for sufficient time to allow the dose to be absorbed.[90]

Medications should not be administered through enteral tubes on free-drainage.[137]

> When a patient who was previously on oral medication has an enteral feeding tube fitted and is likely to have medication administered via this route, contact Pharmacy for advice.

2.2 Problem solving

What do you do if giving several medications?

Do not mix drugs together during preparation, dispersal, or in the syringe. Drugs are more likely to interact with each other if mixed together directly, particularly following tablet crushing. Also if the tube becomes blocked it may be difficult to determine how much of the dose has been given.

Administer each drug separately (see flow chart, section 3.2).

What can be done if the tube becomes blocked?

Adequate tube flushing and appropriate preparation of medications should prevent tube blockage. However if blockage does occur, first aspirate to try and remove any particulate matter, then flush the tube with warm water.[113] Do NOT use excessive force.[112]

Other methods which have been tried include flushing the feeding tube with lemonade, sodium bicarbonate, cola or soda water. The combination of the acidity of these drinks, the effervescence due to carbonation and the flushing action may dislodge the blockage. However some sources consider the use of acidic drinks to contribute to tube blockage through protein denaturation.[119]

Another method involves adding the contents of three Pancrex V capsules and 1g of sodium bicarbonate powder to 20ml distilled water, instilling the solution into the enteral feeding tube and leaving it in the tube for twenty minutes before flushing with distilled water. Both the Pancrex V capsules and the sodium bicarbonate must be prescribed before this method is used.[155]

Are injectable drugs suitable to be used down the tube?

Some injectable drugs are suitable for oral administration and can be given via enteral feeding tubes, e.g. vancomycin, hyoscine. Injections with a high polyethylene glycol content are not suitable for enteral administration.[104] See individual drug monographs for advice.

Is it possible to add medication to the feed?

No, medication must never be added to feeds. Changes in feed rate would alter drug dosage with a risk or under / over-dosing. There is a risk of microbiological contamination of the feed and there are difficulties in predicting the effect the feed will have on the physical characteristics and stability of the medication, and vice versa.

Is it possible to add medication to soft food to aid swallowing?

Sometimes this may be done, but it is usually outside the product licence. When this is done, the medication should be added to the first mouthful of food so that the whole dose is given. Some medications can be added to fruit juice or other fluids for administration. See individual drug monographs for advice. Due to the potential for drug interactions, do not add drugs to grapefruit juice.

2.3 Reasons for unpredictable response

Reason One

Drugs may bind to the enteral feeding tube, resulting in reduced absorption and bioavailability of the drug.

Examples:
- Lansoprazole suspension.
- Carbamazepine suspension.
- Phenytoin suspension.

Reason Two

Nutrients in the enteral feed may increase or decrease absorption of the drug from the stomach. This will consequently affect the drug levels in the body.

- Highly protein bound drugs such as theophylline may interact with the protein content of the feed. This may result in decreased effects.
- Some drugs may be required to be taken on an empty stomach e.g. flucloxacillin, tetracyclines. Tetracyclines may bind to some components of the feed, causing a decrease in the bioavailability of the drug.
- Digoxin interacts with enteral feeds which are high in fibre such as Jevity®.

Reason Three

Diarrhoea can be a problem in post-pyloric feeding. This is partly because the jejunum lacks the reservoir effect provided by the gastric fluids in the stomach and partly because the protective action of the pylorus in the regulation of delivery of nutrients into the intestine is bypassed.[3] Many liquid medications are hyperosmolar or hypertonic, and when administered directly into the jejunum osmotic diarrhoea and nausea can occur.

3. General guidance on administration of medication via enteral feeding tubes

3.1 Review process for patients who have had an enteral feeding tube fitted

Step One

Can the current oral medication be administered by an alternative route?

Other methods of administration

RECTAL	e.g. aspirin, diclofenac, and paracetamol suppositories
PARENTERAL	e.g. intravenous, intramuscular and subcutaneous injections
TRANSDERMAL	e.g. hyoscine, glyceryl trinitrate, and hormone replacement therapy patches
SUBLINGUAL / BUCCAL TABLETS	e.g. prochlorperazine 3mg tablets

Step Two

Can the current oral medication be changed to another medication which has a more suitable method of administration?

e.g. mefenamic acid tablets changed to diclofenac suppositories.
e.g. isosorbide mononitrate tablets changed to glyceryl trinitrate patches.

Step Three

If the medication cannot be changed to an alternate route or medication, does it come as a liquid or as a dispersible / soluble tablet?

When medications have to be given by enteral feeding tube, liquids / dispersible tablets are the preferred formulations. Tablets should only be crushed as a last resort.

Many sugar–free liquids contain sorbitol, an artificial sweetener, which is a laxative and at total daily doses of 7.5g and upwards can result in abdominal cramping and diarrhoea.[116] Sorbitol has a cumulative effect and it is therefore important to minimise the intake of sorbitol where possible. Cost implications occur when the drug is only available in paediatric preparations and large volumes will be required.

Step Four

When changing from solid to liquid dosage forms should any dose changes be made?

If changing from slow release tablets / capsules to liquid it may to necessary to decrease the dose and increase the frequency of administration.

Some drugs have a different bioavailability when being changed from a tablet to a liquid, e.g. digoxin. Other drugs contain a different salt of the drug in the liquid and tablet form, e.g. phenytoin. See recommendations under individual drug monographs, or contact Pharmacy for advice.

Step Five

Does the feeding regimen need to be adjusted?

Many medications interact with enteral feeds. This can result in increased or decreased absorption, altered therapeutic effects and adverse effects, and sometimes blockage of the enteral feeding tube. Medications may have to be given during a feeding break, which may necessitate pausing the enteral feed (and therefore increasing the feed rate at other times to ensure that adequate nutrition is achieved). In order to reduce the number of feed breaks required, drug frequency may have to be adjusted. See recommendations under individual drug monographs.

Contact Pharmacy and the Nutrition team for advice on patient management.

3.2 Medicine administration flow chart
– enteral tubes[112]

Review medication and agree with the prescriber how it is to be given. Contact Pharmacy for advice. If any of the medication has to be given during feeding breaks, consult with the Nutrition team and Pharmacy to rearrange doses and feeding breaks to coincide.

When a dose is due:-

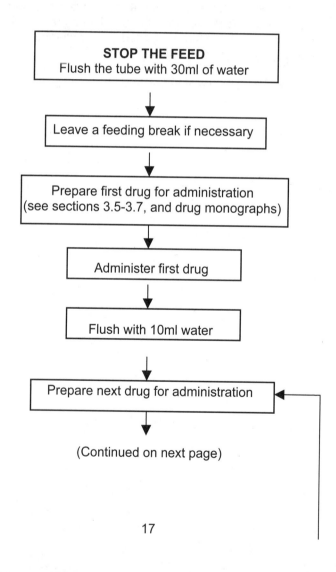

STOP THE FEED
Flush the tube with 30ml of water

Leave a feeding break if necessary

Prepare first drug for administration
(see sections 3.5-3.7, and drug monographs)

Administer first drug

Flush with 10ml water

Prepare next drug for administration

(Continued on next page)

(Continued from previous page)

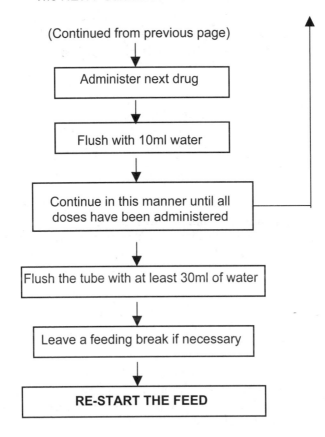

Administer next drug

Flush with 10ml water

Continue in this manner until all doses have been administered

Flush the tube with at least 30ml of water

Leave a feeding break if necessary

RE-START THE FEED

3.3 General guidelines for administration of medications through enteral feeding tubes

Standard tablets
Crushing should be avoided. If crushing is the only option then the tablets should be crushed well enough to prevent clogging of the tube. Care should be taken when crushing drugs which have a high incidence of allergic reactions e.g. antibiotics, chlorpromazine. It is important to ensure that the whole dose is administered.

Dispersible and effervescent formulations
These are low in osmolality and will not cause diarrhoea. Most dispersible and effervescent formulations contain sodium, which may be a problem in sodium restricted patients.

Enteric-coated (e/c) tablets – do not crush
The enteric coating is designed to prevent drug dissolution in the stomach and to promote absorption in the small intestine. If the tablet is crushed and passed down the enteral feeding tube, undesirable side effects may occur. These could include stomach irritation and a decrease in drug effectiveness. When crushed, the tablet will break into small chunks that bind together when moistened and subsequently clog the feeding tube.[4]

Buccal and sublingual tablets – do not crush
Drugs formulated in these dosage forms such as prochlorperazine (Buccastem®) or glyceryl trinitrate are designed not to pass through the stomach in order to avoid the first pass metabolism effects in the liver. If these tablets are passed down the enteral feeding tube, drug effect will be decreased. Buccal and sublingual tablets are suitable to be used as normal in most cases even if a patient becomes nil by mouth, provided that the patient is safe to have tablets held in their mouth, and is still producing normal quantities of saliva.

Modified-release (MR) and controlled release (CR) preparations (also SR, LA, XL, Retard, Once Weekly) – do not crush

These drugs are intended to be released gradually over time, and often have a special coating to enable this. If the tablet is crushed and passed down the enteral feeding tube an increase in the expected peak plasma level may occur. The patient will be initially exposed to significantly higher than normal levels which will increase the chance of side effects. Later, the drug will not last the full dosage interval, resulting in a period with little or no drug present, possibly resulting in loss of control of the patient's condition.

Cytotoxic tablets – do not crush

All staff should avoid contact with cytotoxic drugs. Contact Pharmacy for advice.

Chewable tablets – do not crush

Some of these tablets, e.g. Tegretol® Retard Chewtabs, are formulated so that they are partially absorbed in the mouth.[5] If the tablet is crushed decreased drug absorption will occur.

3.4 General guidelines for administration of medications to patients with swallowing difficulties

Dispersible / effervescent tablets
Dispersible and effervescent tablets can usually be administered to patients with swallowing difficulties in the normal manner. Dispersible and effervescent tablets should not be mixed with fluids other than water unless specifically indicated in the product information or the individual drug monograph, as this would cause administration to be outside the product licence.

Tablets
Crushing tablets to aid administration to patients with swallowing difficulties is almost always outside the product licence. Crushed tablets are often unpalatable, and may sometimes have an anaesthetic effect on the oral mucosa, which can put the patient at risk of burns. Rinsing the mouth with water after administration of tablets may help to reduce this.

Liquids
Liquids are the preferred method of administering medications to patients with swallowing difficulties. Sorbitol-containing preparations can cause diarrhoea when large volumes (and therefore large sorbitol doses) are given.

Capsules
Opening capsules for administration to patients with swallowing difficulties is almost always outside the product licence. The contents of capsules are often unpalatable, and they may have an anaesthetic effect on the oral mucosa, which can put the patient at risk of burns. The capsule shell may provide stability to the medication or protect if from gastric acid.

Modified-release preparations
Using modified-release preparations in patients with swallowing difficulties poses the same problems as using them in patients with enteral feeding tubes. Modified-release tablets should not be crushed, so a conversion to a non-modified-release preparation is necessary, usually requiring a dose decrease and a dosing frequency increase. Some modified-release capsules contain modified-release beads or granules which can be administered in water or on soft food to patients with swallowing difficulties. However there is a risk of giving excessive doses to patients if the beads / granules are crushed prior to swallowing. Therefore this method should only be used where it is the best possible option for a specific patient, and only if the patient has the ability and understanding to be able to swallow the water / soft food without chewing.

3.5 Directions for administration of tablets

> **IMPORTANT!** – Never leave medication drawn up into a syringe unattended. Never give the syringe to someone else to administer to the patient. Accidental intravenous administration of oral / enteral medication drawn up in syringes has led to fatalities.

Dispersible / disintegrating / soluble tablets – enteral tubes

Some tablets may disperse or disintegrate in water without crushing. If this is the case the tablet should be prepared as follows:

1. Place intact tablet into the barrel of a 50ml oral or bladder-tipped syringe.
2. Replace the plunger and draw up 10-15ml of distilled water.
3. Cap the syringe and allow the tablet to dissolve.
4. Shake well and administer dose down the enteral feeding tube.
5. Flush the tube post dose with 10ml of distilled water.

Effervescent tablets – enteral tubes

These tablets will effervesce and disperse when placed in water. The resulting gases need to be allowed to escape. Prepare as follows:

1. Pour 50ml distilled water into a beaker (some tablets require greater volumes of water – see individual monographs for advice).
2. Add the tablet to the water.
3. Wait for the effervescent reaction to finish.
4. Swirl the solution and draw it all up into a 50ml oral or bladder-tipped syringe (in two aliquots if necessary).
5. Administer the dose down the enteral feeding tube.
6. Rinse the beaker with water and administer this also.
7. Flush the tube post dose with 10ml of distilled water.

Dispersible / effervescent tablets – swallowing difficulties

Put the tablet in a beaker of water (sometimes a large volume is required – see individual monographs for details), and wait for the dispersal / effervescent reaction to finish. The patient should drink the solution immediately, and the beaker should then be rinsed with water and this should be drunk also to ensure the whole dose is given.

Tablets suitable for crushing – enteral tubes

Prepare the tablet as follows:

1. Crush the tablet with a pestle and mortar, a tablet crusher, or between two metal spoons.
2. Add the powder to 15-30ml of distilled water and mix well.
3. Draw up the solution into a 50ml oral or bladder-tipped syringe.
4. Administer the dose down the enteral feeding tube.
5. Rinse out the mortar / tablet crusher with distilled water and administer this also.
6. Flush the tube post dose with 10ml of distilled water.

Tablets suitable for crushing – swallowing difficulties

Prepare the tablet as follows:

1. Crush the tablet with a pestle and mortar, a tablet crusher, or between two metal spoons.
2. Add the powder to 15-30ml of distilled water and mix well.
3. Draw up the solution into an oral or bladder-tipped syringe.
4. Administer the dose to the patient.
5. Rinse out the mortar / tablet crusher with distilled water and administer this also.

DON'T

… **crush tablets in plastic containers as the drug may adhere to the plastic.**
… **use boiling water to dissolve tablets as it may affect bioavailability.**
… **leave oral medicines unattended in syringes.**
… **administer any medicine that you have not prepared yourself.**

3.6 Directions for administration of liquids

IMPORTANT! – Never leave medication drawn up into a syringe unattended. Never give the syringe to someone else to administer to the patient. Accidental intravenous administration of oral / enteral medication drawn up in syringes has led to fatalities.

Liquids / solutions – enteral tubes
Liquids are the preferred formulation for administration via enteral feeding tubes. It is usually not necessary to dilute liquid preparations before administration (but see individual monographs for details). Liquids containing sorbitol may cause diarrhoea, therefore the highest strength product appropriate should be used in order to minimise sorbitol dosage. Sorbitol-containing liquids **should** be diluted before administration.

Flush the tube post dose with 10ml of distilled water.

Syrups – enteral tubes
Syrups have viscous and hyperosmolar properties. It is best to dilute the syrup with the same volume of distilled water before administration.

If the syrup is one of several drugs to be administered it is preferable to administer the syrup last.

Flush the tube post dose with 10ml of distilled water.

Suspensions – enteral tubes
The majority of suspensions are suitable for administration via enteral feeding tubes, however some e.g. ispaghula husk (Fybogel®) sachets for suspension, may block the tube. See individual monographs for advice

Flush the tube post dose with 10ml of distilled water.

Liquids / solutions / syrups / suspensions – swallowing difficulties

These are the preferred formulations for administering medications to patients with swallowing difficulties.

Injections

Use of injections via the enteral route is usually an expensive method of administration, and should be done only if there is no other suitable route or formulation. Not all injections are suitable to be given via the enteral route. Some are hypertonic, and some contain ingredients which are unsuitable for enteral administration, e.g. polyethylene glycol.[137] Only do this on the advice of Pharmacy.

Powder injections should be reconstituted with water for injections. All injections should then be diluted with 30-60ml of water before administration to reduce gastrointestinal side effects.[133,137]

Flush the tube post dose with 10ml distilled water.

3.7 Directions for administration of capsules

> **IMPORTANT!** – Never leave medication drawn up into a syringe unattended. Never give the syringe to someone else to administer to the patient. Accidental intravenous administration of oral / enteral medication drawn up in syringes has led to fatalities.

Hard gelatin capsules – enteral tubes
Prepare the capsule as follows:

1. Gently ease open the capsule to release the powder.
2. Tip the powder into a beaker – be sure to obtain all the powder.
3. Mix the powder with 15-30ml of distilled water.
4. Draw up the solution in an oral or bladder-tipped syringe.
5. Administer the solution through the enteral feeding tube.
6. Rinse the beaker with distilled water, and administer this also.
7. Flush the tube post dose with 10ml of distilled water.

Hard gelatin capsules – swallowing difficulties
Prepare the capsule as follows:

1. Gently ease open the capsule to release the powder.
2. Tip the powder into a beaker – be sure to obtain all the powder.
3. Mix the powder with 15-30ml of distilled water.
4. Draw up the solution in an oral or bladder-tipped syringe.
5. Administer the solution to the patient.
6. Rinse the beaker with distilled water, and administer this also.

Modified-release capsules – enteral tubes
Contact Pharmacy for advice. It may be necessary to change to another preparation.

See section on modified-release tablets (section 3.4). Some modified-release capsules can be opened without losing their modified-release properties (see individual monographs for advice). The beads / granules inside are themselves modified-release, and should not be crushed or chewed.

Modified-release capsules – swallowing difficulties
Contact Pharmacy for advice. It may be necessary to convert to a non-modified-release preparation. Some modified-release capsules contain modified-release beads or granules which can be administered in water or on soft food to patients with swallowing difficulties. There is a risk of giving excessive doses if the beads / granules are crushed prior to swallowing. This method should only be used where it is the best possible option for a specific patient, and only if the patient has the ability and understanding to be able to swallow the water / soft food without chewing.

Soft gelatin capsules e.g. nifedipine – enteral tubes

Method one

1. Pinprick one end of the capsule.
2. Drain out the contents with a syringe.
3. Remove the needle from the syringe.*
4. Dilute if necessary (see individual monographs for advice).
5. Administer through the enteral feeding tube.
6. Flush the tube post dose with 10ml of distilled water.

* Take great care when using needles to prepare doses for oral / enteral administration.

Some of the drug may adhere to the soft gelatin capsule, resulting in a smaller dose than intended being given.

Method two

1. Dissolve capsule in 15-30ml of warm (not hot) water.
2. Remove undissolved gelatin.
3. Draw up the solution in an oral or bladder-tipped syringe.
4. Administer the solution through the enteral feeding tube.
5. Flush the tube post dose with 10ml of distilled water.

Soft gelatin capsules e.g. nifedipine – swallowing difficulties

Method one

1. Pinprick one end of the capsule.
2. Drain out the contents with a syringe.
3. Remove the needle from the syringe.*
4. Dilute if necessary (see individual monographs for advice).
5. Administer to the patient.

Take great care when using needles to prepare doses for oral / enteral administration.

Some of the drug may adhere to the soft gelatin capsule, resulting in a smaller dose than intended being given.

Method two

1. Dissolve capsule in 15-30ml of warm (not hot) water.
2. Remove undissolved gelatin.
3. Draw up the solution in an oral or bladder-tipped syringe.
4. Administer the solution to the patient.

DON'T...

... **microwave – this will affect the stability of the medication.**

4. Drug Monographs

Abacavir

Presentation
Film-coated tablets.
Sugar-free oral solution.

Administration – enteral tubes / swallowing difficulties
Use the oral solution.[132] Follow the directions in section 3.6.

Acarbose

Presentation
Tablets.

Administration – NG / PEG tubes / swallowing difficulties
1st choice – Switch to insulin if appropriate.
2nd choice – The tablets can be crushed and mixed with water for administration via nasogastric tube.[140] Follow the directions in section 3.5.

Administration – NJ / PEJ / PEGJ tubes
1st choice – Switch to insulin if appropriate.

The tablets are not suitable to be crushed for administration via enteral tubes ending in the jejunum.[140]

Clinical guidance
Due to its mechanism of action, the use of acarbose may not be appropriate in patients on continuous enteral feeding. Contact the Nutrition team for advice.

Acebutolol

Presentation
Capsules, film-coated tablets.

Administration – enteral tubes / swallowing difficulties
The capsules can be opened, and the contents dispersed in water for administration.[41,105] Follow the directions in section 3.7.

Aceclofenac

Presentation
Film-coated tablets.

Administration – enteral tubes / swallowing difficulties
1st choice – Switch to an alternative drug which has a dispersible, liquid, or rectal form, e.g. diclofenac, ibuprofen.
2nd choice – The tablet can be crushed and mixed with water for administration.[41] Follow the directions in section 3.5.

Clinical guidance
For short term use only as aceclofenac is more irritant to the gastrointestinal tract after being crushed.

Acenocoumarol (Nicoumalone)

Presentation
Tablets.

Administration – enteral tubes / swallowing difficulties
The tablets can be crushed and mixed with water for administration.[105] Follow the directions in section 3.5.

Acetazolamide

Presentation
Tablets.
Slow release capsules.
Injection.

Administration – enteral tubes / swallowing difficulties
1st choice – A suspension with a 7 day expiry can be made by Pharmacy at some centres.[38] Follow the directions in section 3.6.
2nd choice – The standard tablets disperse with a fine sediment.[7,40,41] They disperse in around five minutes.[154] Follow the directions in section 3.5.
3rd choice – The injection can be dissolved in water and used enterally.[40,104,138,152] Follow the directions in section 3.6.

The slow release capsules are not considered suitable for use, although in some centres they have been opened and the contents flushed down enteral feeding tubes.[133] Contact Pharmacy for advice.

Acetylcysteine

Presentation
Effervescent tablets.
Injection.

Administration – enteral tubes / swallowing difficulties
1st choice – Use the effervescent tablets. Follow the directions in section 3.5.
2nd choice – The injection can be diluted 1:4 in orange juice for enteral administration. It has a bitter taste.[40,152] Orange or blackcurrant syrup can also be used to dilute the injection solution.[152]

Feed guidance
Enteral feeds should be stopped prior to administration of acetylcysteine, and restarted afterwards.[158]

Aciclovir

Presentation
Tablets.
Dispersible tablets.
Suspension (contains sorbitol).
Intravenous infusion.

Administration – enteral tubes / swallowing difficulties
1st choice – Give by intravenous infusion.
2nd choice – Use the suspension or the dispersible tablets.[104] Follow the directions in sections 3.5 and 3.6.

Acipimox

Presentation
Capsules.

Clinical guidance
Administration via enteral feeding tube not recommended. Contact Pharmacy for advice.[140]

Acitretin

Presentation
Capsules.

Administration – enteral tubes
The capsule contents are poorly soluble, and are therefore not suitable to be used via enteral feeding tubes as they may cause blockage.[105]

Administration – swallowing difficulties
Caution – teratogenic. Women of childbearing potential must not engage in any activity (i.e. capsule opening) where exposure to this drug may occur.[162]
For patients with swallowing difficulties, the capsules can be opened and their contents sprinkled onto soft food.[105]

Albendazole

Presentation
Tablets (named patient supply).
Suspension (named patient supply).

Administration – enteral tubes
No information about the use of this medication via enteral feeding tubes has been located.

Administration – swallowing difficulties
Use the suspension if available. Some sources advise against crushing the tablets.[41] However this has been done when necessary.[152] Contact Pharmacy for advice.

Alendronic acid

Presentation
Tablets

Clinical guidance
The tablets are not considered suitable for crushing due to the risk of oesophageal damage, although this has been done in some centres and the drug is reported to be soluble.[50,155] (NB The presence of a naso-gastric / jejunal tube compromises the cardiac sphincter and increases the risk of oesophageal damage).

Review whether the medication is still needed. Contact Pharmacy for advice.

Alfacalcidol

Presentation
Capsules.
Oral drops.
Injection.

Administration – enteral tubes
Recommended method - give by parenteral injection.

The oral drops are unstable and not suitable for dilution. They may adsorb onto plastic and therefore should not be given via enteral feeding tubes. Anecdotally the drops have been administered via enteral feeding tubes with effect, but this is not recommended.

Administration – swallowing difficulties
The drops can be administered on a spoon for patients with swallowing difficulties.[128] They are light sensitive.[133] Some sources state that alfacalcidol drops can be mixed with milk prior to administration, however the manufacturers do not recommend this, as studies have suggested that the dose is not reproducible when given in this manner.[128,152]

Alfuzosin

Presentation
Film-coated tablets.
Modified-release tablets.

Administration – enteral tubes / swallowing difficulties
The standard (film-coated) tablets can be crushed and dispersed in water for administration.[42] Follow the directions in section 3.5.

The modified-release tablets should not be crushed. Contact Pharmacy for advice.

Clinical guidance
Monitor blood pressure.

Alimemazine (Trimeprazine)

Presentation
Film-coated tablets.
Syrup.

Administration – enteral tubes / swallowing difficulties
1st choice – Use the syrup.[104] Follow the directions in section 3.6.
2nd choice – The tablets can be crushed and mixed with water for administration. The blue film-coating can be washed off the tablets to make them more easy to crush.[152] Follow the directions in section 3.5.

Allopurinol

Presentation
Tablets.
Sugar-free oral suspension (special).

Administration – enteral tubes / swallowing difficulties
1st choice – Use the oral suspension if available. Follow the directions in section 3.6.
2nd choice – The tablets can be crushed and mixed with water for administration.[8,40] The 100mg tablets will disperse within one minute without crushing.[154] The 300mg tablets must be crushed before dispersing in water.[154] Follow the directions in section 3.5. Give immediately.[155]

Feed guidance
Give after feed.[35]

Aluminium hydroxide

Presentation
Tablets, capsules.
Oral suspension.

Administration – enteral tubes
Not recommended for administration via enteral feeding tubes as it
may interact with enteral feeds to form protein complexes.[104]

Administration – swallowing difficulties
Use the suspension.

Alverine citrate

Presentation
Capsules.

Administration – enteral tubes / swallowing difficulties
The capsules can be opened, and the contents dispersed in water
for administration.[105] Follow the directions in section 3.7. The
capsule contents have an anaesthetic effect.[105]

Amantadine

Presentation
Capsules.
Syrup.

Administration – enteral tubes / swallowing difficulties
Use the syrup (contains sorbitol[104]).[41,104] Follow the directions in
section 3.6.

Amiloride

Presentation
Tablets.
Oral solution.

Administration – enteral tubes / swallowing difficulties
1st choice – Use the oral solution.[104] Follow the directions in section 3.6.
2nd choice – The tablets can be crushed and dispersed in water for administration.[94] Follow the directions in section 3.5.

Aminophylline

Presentation
Tablets.
Modified-release tablets.
Injection.

Clinical guidance
Consider changing to equivalent does of theophylline liquid. Seek advice from Pharmacy.

Amiodarone

Presentation
Tablets.
Concentrate for infusion.

Administration - enteral tubes
1st choice – Give by infusion if appropriate.
2nd choice – A suspension can be made by Pharmacy at some centres. Follow the directions in section 3.6.
3rd choice – The tablets can be crushed and mixed with water for administration.[42,152] Without crushing they disperse in around five minutes.[154] Follow the directions in section 3.5. Give immediately.[7,8]

Administration – swallowing difficulties
1st choice – Give by infusion if appropriate.
2nd choice – A suspension can be made by Pharmacy at some centres. Follow the directions in section 3.6.
3rd choice – The tablets can be crushed and mixed with water for administration.[42,152] Without crushing they disperse in around five minutes.[154] Follow the directions in section 3.5. Give immediately.[7,8]
The crushed tablets have a bitter taste.[105] They can be mixed with fruit juice if desired.[132]

Amisulpride

Presentation
Tablets.
Solution.

Administration - enteral tubes / swallowing difficulties
Use the solution.[132] Follow the directions in section 3.6.

Amitriptyline

Presentation
Tablets.
Oral solution.

Administration - enteral tubes / swallowing difficulties
1st choice – Use the oral solution.[104] Absorption may be decreased by high fibre feeds.[41] Follow the directions in section 3.6.
2nd choice – The tablets can be crushed and dispersed in water.[105]
Follow the directions in section 3.5.

Amlodipine

Presentation
Tablets.

Administration - enteral tubes / swallowing difficulties
The tablet will disperse in water.[7,37,152] They disperse in one to five minutes.[154] Follow the directions in section 3.5. Give immediately as the drug is light sensitive.[104]

Amoxapine

Presentation
Tablets.

Administration - enteral tubes / swallowing difficulties
The tablets can be crushed and mixed with water for administration.[104] Follow the directions in section 3.5.

Amoxicillin (Amoxycillin)

Presentation
Capsules.
Sugar free syrup, suspension, sugar free suspension (some contain sorbitol), sachets.
Injection.

Administration - NG / PEG tubes / swallowing difficulties
1st choice – Give by parenteral injection if appropriate.
2nd choice – Use the syrup or the suspension.[104] Follow the directions in section 3.6.

Administration – NJ / PEJ / PEGJ tubes
1st choice – Give by parenteral injection if appropriate.
2nd choice – Administer the injection, reconstituted with sterile water, via the enteral tube, as the suspension has a high osmolality which may lead to an osmotic diarrhoea.[104,158] It is likely that amoxicillin has a similar absorption following administration directly into the jejunum as it does following oral administration.[158]

Amphotericin

Presentation
Tablets.
Suspension.
Lozenges.
Intravenous infusion.

Administration - enteral tubes / swallowing difficulties
Use intravenous preparations where indicated. For intestinal candidiasis, use the suspension.[40] Follow the directions in section 3.6. When the lozenges are indicated, contact Pharmacy for advice.

Ampicillin

Presentation
Capsules.
Oral suspension.
Injection.

Clinical guidance
Enteral ampicillin is poorly absorbed compared with enteral amoxicillin, so amoxicillin is the preferred antibiotic for enteral administration.[158]

Anastrozole

Presentation
Film-coated tablets.

Administration - enteral tubes / swallowing difficulties
The tablets can be crushed and mixed with water for administration.[46] Follow the directions in section 3.5.

Antacids

Clinical guidance
Aluminium containing antacids may interact with feeds and form a plug.[135] Contact Pharmacy for advice on suitable alternatives.

Arginine

Presentation
Tablets (special).
Solution.
Powder (special).
Injection (special).

Administration – enteral tubes
No information about the use of this medication via enteral feeding tubes has been located.

Administration – swallowing difficulties
Use either the solution or the powder. They may be mixed with milk or fruit juice to improve palatability.[152] The 10% injection has been used orally.[152,160]

Arthrotec®

Presentation
Tablets.

Clinical guidance
The tablets are formed of a core of diclofenac surrounded by a mantle of misoprostol. They are not suitable for crushing.[51] Contact Pharmacy for advice.

Asasantin®

Presentation
Modified-release capsules.

Clinical guidance
The capsules are modified-release and should not be opened. They contain aspirin and dipyridamole. Patients should be converted onto the two component drugs. Contact Pharmacy for advice.

Ascorbic acid

Presentation
Tablets.
Effervescent tablets.
Injection.

Administration - enteral tubes / swallowing difficulties
Use the effervescent tablets if possible.[94,104] Where lower doses are necessary, the effervescent tablets can be halved / quartered and dispersed in water, or the standard tablets can be crushed and mixed with water for administration.[104] Follow the directions in section 3.5.

Aspirin

Presentation
Tablets.
Enteric-coated tablets.
Dispersible tablets.
Suppositories (may not be available).

Administration - enteral tubes / swallowing difficulties
1st choice – Use the suppositories (if available).
2nd choice – Use the dispersible tablets.[104] Give with food.[35] Follow the directions in section 3.5.

Do not crush enteric-coated tablets.

A single case report of aspirin administration directly into the jejunum showed absorption comparable to oral administration.[158]

Atazanavir

Presentation
Capsules.

Administration - enteral tubes
The capsules can be opened and the contents dispersed in water for administration.[132] Follow the directions in section 3.7.

Administration – swallowing difficulties
The capsules can be opened and the contents dispersed in water or mixed with soft food.[132] Follow the directions in section 3.7.

Atenolol

Presentation
Tablets, film-coated tablets.
Syrup (contains sorbitol).
Injection.

Administration - enteral tubes / swallowing difficulties
1st choice – Give by parenteral injection if appropriate.
2nd choice – Use the syrup and protect from light.[40,88] Follow the directions in section 3.6.
3rd choice – The tablets can be crushed and mixed with water for administration.[133] Follow the directions in section 3.5.

Some sources recommend that only the crushed tablets should be used for patients with enteral feeding tubes terminating in the jejunum.[155]

Atorvastatin

Presentation
Film-coated tablets.

Administration - enteral tubes / swallowing difficulties
The tablets can be crushed and mixed with water for administration.[37] Follow the directions in section 3.5. Atorvastatin tablets are not very soluble and a residue may be left, with the potential to block the enteral feeding tube. Flush well after dosing.[37,104]

Atropine sulphate

Presentation
Tablets.
Liquid (special).
Injection.

Administration - enteral tubes / swallowing difficulties
1st choice – Use the liquid.[138] Follow the directions in section 3.6.
2nd choice – The tablets may be crushed and mixed with water for administration.[138] Follow the directions in section 3.5.
3rd choice – The injection has been given enterally.[152] Follow the directions in section 3.6.

Azathioprine

Presentation
Tablets, film-coated tablets.
Injection.
Suspension can be made by Pharmacy.

Clinical guidance
Caution – cytotoxic. Contact Pharmacy for advice before giving.
Give by parenteral injection if appropriate. Alternatively contact
Pharmacy for the suspension. Follow the directions in section 3.6.

The tablet is cytotoxic and should not be crushed or dissolved except
on Pharmacy advice. If no other method is appropriate, on advice
from Pharmacy ONLY the tablet can be dispersed in water for
administration.[155] The drug is light sensitive, so give immediately.[155]

Azithromycin

Presentation
Capsules.
Suspension.

Administration - enteral tubes / swallowing difficulties
Use the suspension.[105] Follow the directions in section 3.6.

Feed guidance
Withhold enteral feeds for two hours before and one hour after each
dose.[152]

Baclofen

Presentation
Liquid.
Tablets.

Administration - enteral tubes / swallowing difficulties
1st choice – Use the liquid. Follow the directions in section 3.6. The liquid may be difficult to use via fine bore tubes as it is quite thick.[132]
2nd choice – The tablets are dispersible.[38,39] Follow the directions in section 3.5.

Balsalazide

Presentation
Capsules.

Administration - enteral tubes / swallowing difficulties
The capsules can be opened, and the contents dispersed in water for administration.[104] The manufacturer advises against this, however, as the contents of the capsules will stain badly.[105] Use an alternative treatment if possible. If not use the capsules, and take care. Follow the directions in section 3.7.

Bendroflumethiazide (Bendrofluazide)

Presentation
Tablets.

Administration - enteral tubes / swallowing difficulties
1st choice – A suspension can be made by Pharmacy at some centres. Follow the directions in section 3.6.
2nd choice – The tablets will disperse readily in water.[38,39,40,41,152] They disperse in one to five minutes.[154] Follow the directions in section 3.5.

Benperidol

Presentation
Tablets.

Administration - enteral tubes / swallowing difficulties
A suspension can be made by Pharmacy in some centres.[138] Follow the directions in section 3.6.

Benzatropine (Benztropine)

Presentation
Tablets (may not be available).
Injection.

Administration - enteral tubes / swallowing difficulties
1st choice – Give by parenteral injection if appropriate.
2nd choice – The tablets can be crushed and mixed with water for administration.[41] Follow the directions in section 3.5.
3rd choice – The injection has also been administered enterally, however the manufacturers cannot recommend this.[104] Follow the directions in section 3.6.

Betahistine

Presentation
Tablets.

Administration - enteral tubes / swallowing difficulties
The tablets can be crushed and mixed with water for administration.[41] Follow the directions in section 3.5.

Betaine

Presentation
Tablets (special).
Powder.
Powder for oral solution (special).

Administration – enteral tubes
No information about the use of this medication via enteral feeding tubes has been located.

Administration – swallowing difficulties
Use the powder for oral solution if available.[15] Follow the directions in section 3.6.

Betamethasone

Presentation
Tablets.
Soluble tablets.
Injection.

Administration - enteral tubes / swallowing difficulties
Use the soluble tablets.[41] Follow the directions in section 3.5.

Bethanechol

Presentation
Tablets.

Administration - enteral tubes / swallowing difficulties
The tablets can be crushed and mixed with water for administration.[105] Follow the directions in section 3.5.

Feed guidance
Withhold enteral feeds for one hour before and one hour after each dose.[136]

Bezafibrate

Presentation
Tablets.
Modified-release tablets.

Administration - enteral tubes / swallowing difficulties
The 200mg (standard) tablet will disperse in water over 1-2 minutes, or can be crushed.[52,154] Follow the directions in section 3.5. If giving via enteral feeding tube, flush well after each dose.

Do not crush the modified-release tablets.[52] Contact Pharmacy for advice on switching patients from the modified-release tablets to the standard tablets.

Bicalutamide

Presentation
Tablets.

Administration - enteral tubes / swallowing difficulties
The tablets are very insoluble but can be crushed finely and mixed with water for administration.[46] Follow the directions in section 3.5.

Biotin

Presentation
Tablets (named patient).
Injection (named patient).

Administration – enteral tubes
No information about the use of this medication via enteral feeding tubes has been located.

Administration – swallowing difficulties
The tablets may be crushed and mixed with a drink.[152]

Bisacodyl

Presentation
Enteric-coated tablets.
Suppositories.

Administration - enteral tubes / swallowing difficulties
Use the suppositories.

The tablet has an enteric coating. Do not crush as it has an irritant effect on the stomach.[41]

Bisoprolol

Presentation
Tablets, film-coated tablets.

Administration - enteral tubes / swallowing difficulties
1st choice – Change to atenolol, which has a syrup formulation. See atenolol monograph and follow the directions in section 3.6.
2nd choice – The tablets can be crushed finely and mixed with water for administration. The lower strength tablets will disperse in one to five minutes without crushing.[154] The higher strength tablets should be crushed before mixing with water.[154] Follow the directions in section 3.5. If giving via enteral feeding tube, flush well after each dose.[95]

Bromocriptine

Presentation
Tablets.
Capsules.

Administration - enteral tubes / swallowing difficulties
The tablets can be dispersed in water for administration.[95] They disperse in one to five minutes.[154] Follow the directions in section 3.5. The drug must be protected from light, so give immediately, and flush well with water.[41]

Brompheniramine

Presentation
Syrup.

Administration - enteral tubes / swallowing difficulties
Use the syrup.[41] Follow the directions in section 3.6.

The liquid is not compatible with feeds, so flush well before and after each dose.[41]

Budesonide

Presentation
Capsules.
Modified-release capsules.
Enema.

Administration – enteral tubes
The capsules can be opened, and the granular contents dispersed in fruit juice for administration.[105] Follow the directions in section 3.7.

Do not open the modified-release capsules for use via feeding tubes. The enema is for rectal use only and may not be suitable for most patients.

Administration – swallowing difficulties
For patients with swallowing difficulties, Entocort® CR capsules have been opened and the pellets mixed with orange juice for administration. The pellets should not be crushed, therefore this method may not be appropriate for patients with limited understanding or impaired ability to follow instructions.[132,138,152]

Bumetanide

Presentation
Sugar-free liquid (contains sorbitol).
Tablets.
Injection.

Administration - enteral tubes / swallowing difficulties
1st choice – Use the liquid. Follow the directions in section 3.6.
2nd choice – The tablet can be crushed and mixed with water for administration.[38,39,154] Follow the directions in section 3.5.

Buprenorphine

Presentation
Sublingual tablets.
Transdermal patches.
Injection.

Administration - enteral tubes / swallowing difficulties
Use the patches or give by parenteral injection if appropriate. If the patient is safe to use the sublingual tablets and has a sufficiently moist mouth, these may continue to be used sublingually.

The sublingual tablets are not suitable to be administered via enteral feeding tube as the drug undergoes extensive first pass metabolism.[141]

Buspirone

Presentation
Tablets.

Administration - enteral tubes / swallowing difficulties
The tablets can be crushed and dispersed in water for administration.[41] Without crushing they disperse in around five minutes.[154] Follow the directions in section 3.5.

Feed guidance
Buspirone plasma concentration may be increased by enteral feeding. The doses should be given at the same time each day in relation to feeding.[155]

Busulfan (Busulphan)

Presentation
Film-coated tablets.
Concentrate for infusion.

Administration - enteral tubes / swallowing difficulties
Caution – cytotoxic. Contact Pharmacy for advice before giving. A suspension can be made by Pharmacy at some centres.[138] Follow the directions in section 3.6.

Cabergoline

Presentation
Tablets.

Administration - enteral tubes / swallowing difficulties
The tablets can be crushed and mixed with water for administration.[105] Follow the directions in section 3.5.

Caffeine

Presentation
Sugar-free oral solution (unlicensed special).
Injection.

Administration - enteral tubes / swallowing difficulties
1st choice – Give by intravenous injection / infusion if appropriate.
2nd choice – Use the oral solution if available. Follow the directions
in section 3.6.

Calcium and Vitamin D

Presentation
Various.

Administration - enteral tubes / swallowing difficulties
Contact Pharmacy for advice on equivalent doses. Consider Cacit
D3 sachets.[132]

Calcium carbonate

Presentation
1.25g (500mg [12.6mmol] calcium) chewable tablets (Calcichew).
1.25g (500mg [12.6mmol] calcium) effervescent tablets (Cacit).

Administration - enteral tubes / swallowing difficulties
Use the effervescent tablets. The chewable tablets should not be
used.[94] Follow the directions in section 3.5.

Calcium folinate

Presentation
Tablets.
Injection.

Administration - enteral tubes / swallowing difficulties
1st choice – Give by parenteral injection if appropriate.
2nd choice – The tablets can be dispersed in water for administration.[40] They disperse immediately.[154] Follow the directions in section 3.5.
3rd choice – The injection can be given enterally.[152] Follow the directions in section 3.6.

Calcium glubionate and lactobionate

Presentation
108.3mg [2.7mmol] in 5ml syrup (Calcium-Sandoz).

Administration - enteral tubes / swallowing difficulties
Use the syrup.[104] Follow the directions in section 3.6.

Calcium gluconate

Presentation
600mg (53.4mg [1.35mmol] calcium) tablets.
1g (89mg [2.25mmol] calcium) effervescent tablets.
Injection.

Administration - enteral tubes / swallowing difficulties
Use the effervescent tablets.[40,41] Follow the directions in section 3.5.

Feed guidance
Give during a feeding break (hold enteral feeds for one hour before and one hour after dose).[41]

Calcium resonium

Presentation
Powder for oral administration.
Enemas.

Administration - enteral tubes / swallowing difficulties
Use the enemas rectally.[105]

The powder for oral administration should not be given via enteral feeding tubes due to the risk of tube blockage.[105]

Candesartan

Presentation
Tablets.

Administration - enteral tubes / swallowing difficulties
The tablets can be crushed and mixed with water for administration.[53] Without crushing they disperse in around five minutes.[154] Follow the directions in section 3.5. No information is available on whether candesartan is likely to block enteral feeding tubes.[53]

Captopril

Presentation
Tablets.
Liquid (special[150]).
Liquid can be made by Pharmacy.

Administration - enteral tubes / swallowing difficulties
1st choice – A liquid can be prepared by Pharmacy at some centres. Follow the directions in section 3.6.
2nd choice – The tablets will disperse in water in one to five minutes.[7,39,40,152,154] Follow the directions in section 3.5. A fine powder sediment may be left, so if giving via enteral feeding tube, flush well after each dose.[104]

Clinical guidance
Captopril tablets have been given sublingually. To use this route, the dose should be halved and given twice as frequently, i.e. 25mg twice daily becomes 12.5mg four times daily.[105] Monitor blood pressure.

Feed guidance
Give on an empty stomach. Withhold enteral feeds for at least half an hour before and half an hour after each dose.

Carbamazepine

Presentation
Tablets.
Chewtabs.
Liquid.
Suppositories.
Modified-release tablets.

Administration - enteral tubes
1st choice – Use the suppositories if possible. They are licensed for a maximum of seven days, at a maximum dose of 1g/day.[35]
2nd choice – Use the liquid (contains sorbitol[104]), and dilute with an equal volume of water before administration.[104] Follow the directions in section 3.6.

Administration – swallowing difficulties
Use the suppositories or the liquid (contains sorbitol[104]).

Clinical guidance
If changing from Retard formulations to liquid preparation give the same daily dose but increase the frequency of administration. Consider monitoring drug levels when doses have been changed or if there is concern about under / over-dosing.

Carbamazpine MR tablet 400mg twice a day	equivalent to	Carbamazepine liquid 200mg four times a day
100mg tablet / liquid	equivalent to	125mg suppository[90]

Carbamazepine is absorbed onto PVC feeding tubes. However it has been shown that when the suspension is diluted with an equal volume of water, loss is negligible.[10]

Feed guidance
Carbamazepine is slowly and irregularly absorbed from the gastrointestinal tract.[9] Care must be taken to administer carbamazepine at the same time and in the same manner each day so that variations in the extent of drug absorption are minimised. Stop enteral feeds for at least two hours before and two hours after dose to maximise drug absorption.[104]

Carbamylglutamate

Presentation
Dispersible tablets.

Administration - enteral tubes / swallowing difficulties
Use the dispersible tablets.[152] Follow the directions in section 3.5.

Carbimazole

Presentation
Tablets.
Suspension (special[150,155]).

Administration - enteral tubes / swallowing difficulties
The tablets can be crushed and dispersed in water for
administration.[95] Follow the directions in section 3.5.

Carbocisteine

Presentation
Capsules.
Liquid.

Administration - enteral tubes / swallowing difficulties
Use the liquid.[41] Follow the directions in section 3.6.

Carvedilol

Presentation
Tablets.

Administration - enteral tubes / swallowing difficulties
The tablets can be dispersed to form a suspension in water.[52] They
disperse in one to five minutes.[154] Follow the directions in section
3.5. Use immediately.[52]

Cefadroxil

Presentation
Capsules.
Suspension.

Administration - enteral tubes / swallowing difficulties
Use the suspension.[94] Follow the directions in section 3.6.

Cefalexin (Cephalexin)

Presentation
Capsules.
Tablets.
Suspension, syrup.

Administration - enteral tubes / swallowing difficulties
Use the suspension.[104] Follow the directions in section 3.6.

Clinical guidance
There may be reduced absorption when administered directly into the jejunum.[104,137,158] The suspension is hyperosmolar, and may also cause diarrhoea when administered in the jejunum.[155] Dilute well before administration.

Cefixime

Presentation
Film-coated tablets.
Suspension.

Administration - enteral tubes / swallowing difficulties
Use the suspension.[41] Follow the directions in section 3.6.

Cefpodoxime

Presentation
Film-coated tablets.
Suspension.

Administration - enteral tubes / swallowing difficulties
Use the suspension.[79] Follow the directions in section 3.6.

Cefradine (Cephradine)

Presentation
Capsules.
Suspension.
Injection.

Administration - enteral tubes / swallowing difficulties
1st choice – Give by parenteral injection if appropriate.
2nd choice – Use the suspension.[41] Follow the directions in section 3.6.

Cefuroxime

Presentation
Film-coated tablets.
Suspension, sachets.
Injection.

Administration – NG / PEG tubes / swallowing difficulties
1st choice – Give by parenteral injection if appropriate.
2nd choice – For patients with enteral tubes terminating in the stomach, use the suspension.[41] Follow the directions in section 3.6. The suspension may be too viscous to administer via fine bore tubes, in which case use the 3rd choice.
3rd choice – For patients with enteral tubes terminating in the stomach, the tablets have been crushed and dispersed in water.[138] Follow the directions in section 3.5.

Administration – NJ / PEJ / PEGJ tubes
1st choice – Give by parenteral injection if appropriate.

Cefuroxime is not suitable to be administered via enteral feeding tubes terminating in the jejunum as absorption is reduced.[155]

Celecoxib

Presentation
Capsules.

Clinical guidance
The capsule should not be opened as it provides some stability to the medication.[54] Contact Pharmacy for advice.

Celiprolol

Presentation
Tablets.

Administration - enteral tubes / swallowing difficulties
The tablets can be dispersed in water for administration.[55] They disperse in one to five minutes.[154] Follow the directions in section 3.5. Some brands of tablet are film coated, so crush finely if giving via enteral feeding tube or the coating may block the tube.[55]

Cetirizine

Presentation
Tablets.
Oral solution.

Administration - enteral tubes / swallowing difficulties
Use the oral solution.[94,104] Follow the directions in section 3.6.

Chenodeoxycholic acid

Presentation
Capsules (named patient).

Administration – enteral tubes
No information about the use of this medication via enteral feeding tubes has been located.

Administration – swallowing difficulties
A suspension can be prepared by adding the contents of one 250mg capsule to 25ml of sodium bicarbonate solution 8.4% (1mmol/ml). This should be used immediately.[152]

Chloral hydrate

Presentation
Tablets (cloral betaine).
Elixir.

Administration - enteral tubes / swallowing difficulties
Use the elixir.[41,104] It is light sensitive, so give immediately.[41] Follow the directions in section 3.6.

Liquid dosage	=	15-45ml with water or milk at bedtime.[106]

Chlorambucil

Presentation
Film-coated tablets.

Administration - enteral tubes / swallowing difficulties
Caution – cytotoxic. Contact Pharmacy for advice before giving.
A suspension can be made by Pharmacy at some centres.[138] Follow the directions in section 3.6.

Chloramphenicol

Presentation
Capsules.
Injection.

Administration - enteral tubes / swallowing difficulties
1st choice – Give by parenteral injection if possible.
2nd choice – Open the capsules and mix the contents with water.[133]
Follow the directions in section 3.7.

Chlordiazepoxide

Presentation
Tablets, capsules.

Administration - enteral tubes / swallowing difficulties
1st choice – Use an alternative agent available for administration by a non-enteral route if possible (e.g. diazepam).
2nd choice – Open the capsules and mix the contents with water.[104]
Follow the directions in section 3.7.

The tablets have been crushed in some centres,[132] but this is not recommended.

Chloroquine

Presentation
250mg chloroquine phosphate (155mg chloroquine base) tablets.
200mg chloroquine sulphate (150mg chloroquine base) film-coated tablets.
68mg/5ml chloroquine sulphate (50mg/5ml chloroquine base) syrup.
54.5mg/ml chloroquine sulphate (40mg/ml chloroquine base) injection.

Administration - enteral tubes / swallowing difficulties
1st choice – Use the syrup.[41] Follow the directions in section 3.6.
2nd choice - The tablets can be crushed and dispersed in water for administration.[105,152] They should be crushed well to ensure that the film coating is broken up. Without crushing they will disperse in one to five minutes.[154] Follow the directions in section 3.5. Protect from light.[41]

The liquid should not be given at the same time as antacids. Chloroquine has a very bitter taste.[79]

Chlorothiazide

Presentation
Tablets.
Suspension.

Administration - enteral tubes / swallowing difficulties
1st choice – Use the suspension. Follow the directions in section 3.6.
2nd choice – The tablet can be crushed and dispersed in water for administration.[7,40] Follow the directions in section 3.5.

Chlorphenamine (Chlorpheniramine)

Presentation
Tablets.
Syrup, oral solution.
Injection.

Administration - enteral tubes / swallowing difficulties
1st choice – Give by parenteral injection if appropriate.
2nd choice – Use the syrup.[40,94,104] Protect from light.[41] Follow the directions in section 3.6.
3rd choice – The injection can be given enterally.[40,164] Follow the directions in section 3.6.

Chlorpromazine

Presentation
Coated tablets.
Syrup, oral solution, suspension (some contain sorbitol).
Injection.
Suppositories (unlicensed).

Administration - enteral tubes / swallowing difficulties
1st choice – Use the suppositories if possible. A dose adjustment is necessary, contact Pharmacy for advice.
2nd choice – Use the oral solution.[94,104] Follow the directions in section 3.6.

Carers should avoid direct contact with chlorpromazine as contact sensitisation may occur.[132] Therefore the tablets should not be crushed.

100mg (base) suppository = 40-50mg (hydrochloride) tablet.[136]

Chlortalidone (Chlorthalidone)

Presentation
Tablets.

Administration - enteral tubes / swallowing difficulties
The tablets will disperse in water.[7,40] They disperse immediately.[154] Follow the directions in section 3.5. A fine powder sediment may be left, so if giving via enteral feeding tube, flush the tube well with water after administration.[104]

Ciclosporin (Cyclosporin)

Presentation
Capsules.
Oral solution.
Concentrate for infusion.

Administration - enteral tubes
Administer ciclosporin oral solution. Do not flush with water after administering the ciclosporin solution but use the same volume of orange juice instead.

Administration – swallowing difficulties
Administer ciclosporin oral solution. The solution may be mixed with orange or apple juice to improve taste.[104]

Clinical guidance
Due to the oily component of the ciclosporin solution, adherence to enteral feeding tubes may occur and subtherapeutic doses are likely. Monitor drug levels closely.

Dose equivalence depends on which brand of ciclosporin was used previously. Contact Pharmacy for advice.

Feed guidance
When giving via enteral feeding tube, leave a time gap of one hour before administering the next drug down the tube.

Cilazapril

Presentation
Film-coated tablets.

Administration - enteral tubes / swallowing difficulties
The tablets can be crushed and mixed with water for administration.[105] Follow the directions in section 3.5.

Cimetidine

Presentation
Tablets.
Syrup.
Injection.

Administration - enteral tubes / swallowing difficulties
1st choice – Consider giving by parenteral injection.
2nd choice – Use the syrup, diluted with an equal amount of water before administration.[133] Follow the directions in section 3.6.
3rd choice – The injection is suitable to be given enterally.[40,158] Follow the directions in section 3.6.

There may be reduced absorption when cimetidine is administered directly into the jejunum.[104,158]

Feed guidance
Cimetidine syrup is incompatible with feeds so allow an enteral feeding gap of one hour before and one hour after each dose.[41]

Cinnarizine

Presentation
Tablets.
Capsules.

Administration - enteral tubes / swallowing difficulties
The tablets can be dispersed in water for administration.[41,95] They disperse within one minute.[154] Follow the directions in section 3.5.
The capsules have been opened in some centres.[133] Follow the directions in section 3.7.

Ciprofibrate

Presentation
Tablets.

Administration - enteral tubes / swallowing difficulties
The tablets can be crushed and mixed with water for administration.[104,105] Follow the directions in section 3.5.

Ciprofloxacin

Presentation
Tablets.
Intravenous infusion.
Suspension.

Administration – enteral tubes
1st choice – Give by parenteral infusion.
2nd choice – The tablets will disperse in water.[7,40,43] The 250mg tablets disperse in one to five minutes.[154] The 500mg tablets disperse in around five minutes.[154] Follow the directions in section 3.5. Flush the enteral tube after each dose with 65ml deionised water.

Do not use the suspension, as it may block the enteral tube.[43]

Administration – swallowing difficulties
Always use the suspension for patients with swallowing difficulties as the crushed tablets have an extremely unpleasant taste.[43]

Clinical guidance
Tap water is not suitable to use, as minerals in the tap water may bind with ciprofloxacin and decrease the amount of drug absorbed.[36] Use doses at the higher end of the normal range in order to compensate for lower absorption.[94]

Ciprofloxacin is believed to be absorbed in the duodenum[15] and not in the jejunum, therefore higher doses should be used if administered through an enteral tube terminating in the jejunum.[158] Contact Pharmacy for advice.

Feed guidance
Ciprofloxacin interacts with enteral feeds to produce insoluble chelates[11,12] and the absorption of the drug is significantly reduced. This may be particularly significant when administered directly in the jejunum.[155] A feeding break of one hour before and two hours after the administration of ciprofloxacin via any type of enteral feeding tube is recommended.[13] It has been shown that the absorption is reduced by 28% when administered with Ensure® and by 33% when administered with Osmolite®.[14]

Citalopram

Presentation
Tablets.
Oral drops.

Administration - enteral tubes / swallowing difficulties
1st choice – Use the drops. The bottle should be inverted, and the drops will flow automatically, - do not shake the bottle. The required number of drops should be mixed with water, orange juice, or apple juice before administration.[123]

8mg (4 drops) of the oral drops = 10mg tablet.[93]

2nd choice – The tablets have been crushed and dispersed in water if the drops are unavailable, but they may taste unpleasant.[132] Follow the directions in section 3.5. If giving via enteral feeding tube, flush well following administration.[155]

Clarithromycin

Presentation
Tablets.
Suspension.
Intravenous infusion.

Administration - enteral tubes
1st choice – Give by intravenous infusion if possible.
2nd choice – The suspension is viscous and may block the tube. If the suspension has to be used, dilute the dose with the same volume of water immediately prior to administration.[56] Follow the directions in section 3.6.

Do not dilute the suspension beyond manufacturer's recommendations until administration, as dilution of the preservative will occur, affecting the expiry of the product.[56]

Administration – swallowing difficulties
Give by intravenous infusion or use the suspension.

Clindamycin

Presentation
Capsules.
Suspension (unlicensed).
Injection.

Administration – enteral tubes
1st choice – Give by parenteral injection if appropriate.
2nd choice – Use the suspension if available.[138] Follow the directions in section 3.6.
3rd choice – The capsules can be opened and the contents dispersed in water.[57] Give immediately. Follow the directions in section 3.7.

Administration – swallowing difficulties
Use the suspension if available. The capsule contents taste extremely unpleasant and may be unpalatable for oral administration in patients with swallowing difficulties.[57] The capsule contents have been mixed with grape juice or maple syrup.[132]

Clobazam

Presentation
Tablets.

Administration - enteral tubes / swallowing difficulties
The tablets can be dispersed in water for administration.[105] They disperse in one to five minutes.[154] Follow the directions in section 3.5. The crushed / dispersed tablets taste unpleasant.[132]

Clomethiazole (Chlormethiazole)

Presentation
Capsules.
Syrup.

Administration – enteral tubes
The syrup interacts with enteral feeding tubes, and should not be used for patients with enteral tubes in situ.[41] Contact Pharmacy for advice.

Administration – swallowing difficulties
Use the syrup.

Clomipramine

Presentation
Capsules.
Modified-release tablets.
Liquid.

Administration - enteral tubes / swallowing difficulties
1st choice – Use the liquid.[104] Follow the directions in section 3.6.
2nd choice – The capsules can be opened, and the contents dispersed in water for administration.[104] Follow the directions in section 3.7.

Do not crush the modified-release tablets.

Clonazepam

Presentation
Tablets.
Oral drops (unlicensed).
Oral solution (unlicensed).
Injection.

Administration – enteral tubes
1st choice – The tablets can be dispersed in at least 30ml of water for administration.[7,40,94,104] They disperse within one minute.[154] Use at least 30ml of water to disperse the tablets in to prevent binding to the enteral tube.[132] Follow the directions in section 3.5.
2nd choice – The injection can be given enterally after dilution with 1ml Water for Injections.[40,152] Follow the directions in section 3.6.

Administration – swallowing difficulties
For patients with swallowing difficulties, use the oral drops or the solution. Do not mix the drops or the solution with water or any other diluent as this may cause the drug to precipitate out.[105]

Clonidine

Presentation
Tablets.
Transdermal plasters (unlicensed).
Injection.

Administration - enteral tubes / swallowing difficulties
1st choice – The injection can be administered orally / via enteral feeding tubes.[100] The injection can either be given neat, or diluted with water prior to administration.[130] The manufacturers have data to suggest that when prepared aseptically, injection diluted with water is stable for 7 days. The injection is tasteless, but if desired it can be mixed with fruit juice for oral administration.[130]
2nd choice – The tablets have been crushed in some centres[132,152], although there is little information available on this. Follow the directions in section 3.5.

The transdermal plasters are indicated for the management of hypertension. However onset of action takes 2-3 days, and so these are probably only suitable when the period for which the patient needs them can be planned for, or is prolonged.[96]

Clopidogrel

Presentation
Tablets.

Administration - enteral tubes / swallowing difficulties
The tablets can be dispersed in water for administration.[42] They disperse in one to five minutes.[154] Follow the directions in section 3.5.

Clozapine

Presentation
Tablets.

Administration - enteral tubes / swallowing difficulties
1st choice – A suspension can be prepared by Pharmacy at some centres.[138] Follow the directions in section 3.6.
2nd choice – The tablets have been crushed and mixed with water for administration.[105] This is not recommended, however. The powder is not soluble.[132] Contact Pharmacy for advice.

Co-amilofruse

Presentation
Tablets.

Administration - enteral tubes / swallowing difficulties
1st choice – Give the components (furosemide and amiloride) separately as both are available as liquids. Follow the directions in section 3.6.
2nd choice – The tablets can be dispersed in water for administration.[39,40] They disperse within one minute.[154] Follow the directions in section 3.5.

Co-amilozide

Presentation
Tablets.

Administration - enteral tubes / swallowing difficulties
The tablets can be crushed and dispersed in water for administration.[105] Most brands disperse immediately.[154] Follow the directions in section 3.5.

Co-amoxiclav

Presentation
Tablets.
Dispersible tablets (250/125).
Suspension (125/31, 250/62, 400/57).
Injection.

Administration - enteral tubes / swallowing difficulties
1st choice – Give by parenteral injection / infusion.
2nd choice – Use the dispersible tablets. Follow the directions in section 3.5.
3rd choice – Use the suspension and dilute with an equal volume of water before administration to avoid "caking".[94,104] Follow the directions in section 3.6.

Administration – swallowing difficulties
Give by parenteral injection / infusion, or use the suspension.

Clinical guidance
The tablets cannot be directly converted to suspension. The proportions of the two drugs in the medication (amoxicillin and clavulanic acid) are different in the two preparations. Always use the equivalent dosage of amoxicillin – i.e. 250mg/125mg tablet is equivalent to 250mg/62mg suspension. Contact Pharmacy for advice.

Co-beneldopa (Madopar)

Presentation
Capsules.
Dispersible tablets.
Modified-release capsules.

Administration - enteral tubes / swallowing difficulties
Use the dispersible tablets. Follow the directions in section 3.5.

Do not open either type of the capsules (modified-release or standard).[104]

Clinical guidance
Dispersible tablets have a faster onset of action and shorter duration of action than modified-release capsules and a direct substitution cannot occur. Contact Pharmacy for advice on dosage conversion.

If changing from capsules to dispersible tablets a direct changeover is acceptable, but the patient should be monitored for any change in effect as there may be an altered bioavailability.

Levodopa is mainly absorbed in the jejunum. Drug effect may be particularly unpredictable in patients with enteral tubes terminating in the jejunum.[155]

Feed guidance
Co-beneldopa's absorption may be enhanced by interactions with enteral feed proteins. To reduce fluctuations in effect, doses should be given at the same time each day in relation to the feed regimen.[135]

Co-careldopa (Sinemet®)

Presentation
Tablets.
Modified-release tablets.

Administration - enteral tubes / swallowing difficulties
The standard Sinemet® tablets will disperse in water for administration down enteral feeding tubes,[49] or the patient can be converted onto co-beneldopa dispersible tablets. Contact Pharmacy for advice. Lower strengths disperse within one minute.[154] The 25/250 strength disperse in one to five minutes.[154] Follow the directions in section 3.5. Give immediately as the drug will oxidise (degrade).[49] A suspension can be made by Pharmacy on request.[155]

Do not crush the modified-release (CR) tablets.

Conversion table[35]

Sinemet® (co-careldopa)	Madopar® (co-beneldopa)
Sinemet® 62.5mg tablet	Madopar® 62.5mg disp. tablet
Sinemet® 110mg tablet	Madopar® 125mg disp. tablet
Sinemet® Plus 125mg tablet	Madopar® 125mg disp. tablet
Sinemet® 275mg tablet	2 x Madopar® 125mg disp. tablet
Half Sinemet® CR 125mg tablet	Seek advice from Pharmacy
Sinemet® CR 250mg tablet	Seek advice from Pharmacy

Clinical guidance
A direct dose conversion may not be appropriate in all patients. Switching to Madopar® 62.5mg given up to four times a day as required by symptoms, then adjusted upwards according to patient requirements and toleration, may be more suitable for some patients.

Levodopa is mainly absorbed in the jejunum. Drug effect may be particularly unpredictable in patients with enteral tubes terminating in the jejunum.[155]

Feed guidance
Absorption of co-careldopa may be altered by enteral feed proteins. To reduce fluctuations in effect, doses should be given at the same time each day in relation to the feed regimen.[135]

Co-codamol

Presentation
Tablets.
Effervescent tablets, sachets.
Capsules.

Administration - enteral tubes / swallowing difficulties
Use the effervescent tablets or the sachets.[94,104] Follow the directions in section 3.5. Consider switching to paracetamol liquid / suppositories with or without codeine syrup or a parenteral opiate if the high sodium load of the effervescent tablets is a problem.

Co-danthramer

Presentation
Capsules.
Suspension.

Administration - enteral tubes / swallowing difficulties
Use the suspension.[104] Follow the directions in section 3.6.

Codeine

Presentation
Tablets.
Syrup, linctus, paediatric linctus.
Injection.

Administration - enteral tubes / swallowing difficulties
Use the syrup or the linctus (contain alcohol).[40,94,104] Dilute with water before administration.[132] Follow the directions in section 3.6.

Co-dydramol

Clinical guidance
Contact Pharmacy for advice on suitable alternatives.

Co-fluampicil

Presentation
Capsules.
Syrup.
Injection.

Administration - enteral tubes / swallowing difficulties
1st choice – Give by parenteral injection.
2nd choice – Use the syrup.[133] Follow the directions in section 3.6.

Colchicine

Presentation
Tablets.

Administration - enteral tubes / swallowing difficulties
The tablets can be dispersed in water for administration.[104,105] They disperse within one minute.[154] Follow the directions in section 3.5.

Colestyramine (Cholestyramine)

Presentation
Sachets.

Administration - enteral tubes / swallowing difficulties
Use the sachets. Follow the directions in section 3.6.

If giving via enteral feeding tube, flush well after each dose.[41]

Clinical guidance
Colestyramine affects the absorption of other medicines, so give all other medicines at least one hour before or four-six hours after a dose of colestyramine.

Combivir

Presentation
Film-coated tablets.

Administration - enteral tubes / swallowing difficulties
1st choice – change to the separate components (zidovudine and lamivudine).
2nd choice – place Combivir tablets in 50ml tepid (not hot) water and allow to dissolve. It has a bitter taste which can be disguised with juice for patients with swallowing difficulties.[132]

Co-phenotrope

Presentation
Tablets.

Administration - enteral tubes / swallowing difficulties
The tablets can be crushed and dispersed in water for administration.[105,152] Follow the directions in section 3.5.

Co-tenidone

Presentation
Tablets.

Administration - enteral tubes / swallowing difficulties
The tablets can be crushed and dispersed in water for administration.[58] Follow the directions in section 3.5. Use immediately.[58]

Co-triamterzide

Presentation
Tablets.

Administration - enteral tubes / swallowing difficulties
The tablets can be crushed and dispersed in water for administration.[7,94,105] Follow the directions in section 3.5.

Co-trimoxazole

Presentation
Tablets.
Suspension.
Solution for injection.

Administration - enteral tubes
Use the suspension (contains sorbitol) and dilute with an equal volume of water before administration.[40,104,133] Follow the directions in section 3.6.

Administration – swallowing difficulties
Use the suspension (contains sorbitol).

Cyclizine

Presentation
Tablets.
Injection.

Administration - enteral tubes / swallowing difficulties
1st choice – Give by parenteral injection.
2nd choice – Switch to an alternative anti-emetic which is available as a liquid or suppositories, e.g. metoclopramide, domperidone.
3rd choice – A suspension can be prepared by Pharmacy at some centres.[155] Follow the directions in section 3.6.
4th choice – The tablets can be crushed and dispersed in water for administration.[41,95,152] Follow the directions in section 3.5. Protect from light.[41] The crushed tablets have a bitter taste.[105]

The injection has also been given enterally in some centres, however the manufacturers have no information on this, and cannot recommend it.[133,165] Contact Pharmacy for advice.

Cyclophosphamide

Presentation
Sugar-coated tablets.
Injection.

Administration - enteral tubes / swallowing difficulties
Caution – cytotoxic. Contact Pharmacy for advice before giving.
1st choice – Consider giving by parenteral injection.
2nd choice – A suspension can be prepared in Pharmacy in some centres.[138,139,172] Follow the directions in section 3.6.
3rd choice – The injection has been used enterally in some centres.[143,172] Contact Pharmacy for advice before doing this.

Cyproterone

Presentation
Tablets.

Administration - enteral tubes / swallowing difficulties
The tablets can be dispersed in water for administration.[40,59] They
disperse in one to two minutes.[154] Follow the directions in section
3.5. No information has been located on whether cyproterone is
likely to block enteral tubes, or on the effect crushing the tablets may
have on absorption.[59]

Dantrolene

Presentation
Capsules.
Injection.

Administration - enteral tubes / swallowing difficulties
The capsules can be opened, and the contents dispersed in water or
acidic fruit juice (e.g. orange[132]) for administration.[104,105] Follow the
directions in section 3.7.

Use of the injection enterally is NOT recommended, as the drug may
hydrolyse in the stomach. The injection formulation also contains
mannitol. It is designed for its licensed indication, malignant
hyperthermia, and is not a substitute for the oral preparation.[166]

Dapsone

Presentation
Tablets.

Administration - enteral tubes / swallowing difficulties
The tablets can be crushed and dispersed in plenty of water for
administration.[104,152] Follow the directions in section 3.5. Protect
from light.[41]

Deflazacort

Presentation
Tablets.

Administration - enteral tubes / swallowing difficulties
The tablets can be dispersed in water for administration.[105] They disperse within one minute.[154] Follow the directions in section 3.5.

Demeclocycline

Presentation
Capsules.

Administration - enteral tubes / swallowing difficulties
A suspension can be prepared by Pharmacy. Follow the directions in section 3.6.

Do not open the capsules as the contents do not disperse in water, and this has led to enteral tube blockage. The capsule contents may cause severe irritation to the mucosa, so they should not be opened for administration to patients with swallowing difficulties either.[155]

Feed guidance
Demeclocycline absorption is reduced by calcium in enteral feeds. Withhold enteral feeds for one hour before and two hours after each dose.[155]

Desferrioxamine

Presentation
Injection.

Administration - enteral tubes / swallowing difficulties
The injection can be given orally or via nasogastric tube in 50-100ml water. It has an unpleasant taste.[152] No information has been located about the administration of desferrioxamine via other types of enteral feeding tube.

Desmopressin

Presentation
Tablets.
Nasal spray, intranasal solution.
Injection.

Administration - enteral tubes / swallowing difficulties
1st choice – Use the nasal route if appropriate.
2nd choice – The tablets can be crushed and mixed with water for administration.[104,105] Follow the directions in section 3.5.

Dexamethasone

Presentation
Tablets.
Oral solution (contains sorbitol).
Injection.

Administration - enteral tubes / swallowing difficulties
1st choice – Give by parenteral injection if appropriate.
2nd choice – Use the oral solution. Follow the directions in section 3.6.
3rd choice – The tablets have been crushed and mixed with water for administration.[94,152] Follow the directions in section 3.5.
4th choice – The injection has been used enterally.[40,152] Follow the directions in section 3.6.

Diazepam

Presentation
Tablets.
Syrup, oral solution (contain sorbitol).
Injection solution, injection emulsion.
Rectal tubes, suppositories.

Administration - enteral tubes / swallowing difficulties
1st choice – Give by intravenous or rectal route. Contact Pharmacy for advice on equivalent dosage.
2nd choice – Use the syrup or the oral solution, (when giving via enteral feeding tube, dilute with water before administration to reduce viscosity and tube binding[132]). Follow the directions in section 3.6.

The injection has also been given enterally in some centres, however the manufacturers have no information on this, and cannot recommend it.[40,167] Contact Pharmacy for advice.

Clinical guidance
If diazepam is administered through long PVC tubes, drug loss may occur as diazepam is significantly adsorbed onto (portex) PVC.[9,12]
Diazepam may also contribute towards blockage of tubes.

Diazoxide

Presentation
Tablets.
Injection.

Administration - enteral tubes / swallowing difficulties
A suspension has been made by Pharmacy in some centres.[138]
Follow the directions in section 3.6.

Diclofenac sodium

Presentation
Enteric-coated tablets.
Dispersible tablets.
Sugar-free oral suspension (special).
Modified-release tablets, modified-release capsules.
Suppositories.
Injection.
Topical gel.

Administration - enteral tubes / swallowing difficulties
1st choice – Give by parenteral injection or use the suppositories for acute situations.
2nd choice – Use the dispersible tablets or the oral suspension.[94,104,105] Follow the directions in sections 3.5 and 3.6.

Do not crush / open the enteric-coated or the modified-release preparations.

Dicycloverine (Dicyclomine)

Presentation
Tablets.
Syrup.

Administration - enteral tubes / swallowing difficulties
1st choice – Use the syrup.[41] Follow the directions in section 3.6.
2nd choice – The tablets may crushed and mixed with water for administration.[152] Follow the directions in section 3.5.

Didanosine

Presentation
Tablets, capsules.

Administration - enteral tubes / swallowing difficulties
The tablets can be crushed and dispersed in water for administration.[132,152] Follow the directions in section 3.5.

Feed guidance
Withhold enteral feeds for one hour before and one hour after each dose.[136]

Digoxin

Presentation
Tablets.
Elixir.
Injection.

Administration - enteral tubes / swallowing difficulties
1st choice – Consider giving by parenteral injection. Contact Pharmacy for advice on appropriate doses.
2nd choice – Use the elixir.[41] Follow the directions in section 3.6.
3rd choice – Use crushed tablets for patients with enteral feeding tubes delivering to the jejunum if osmotic diarrhoea is a problem.[104,158] Follow the directions in section 3.5.

The injection has also been given enterally in some centres, but this is not recommended as bioavailability is unpredictable.[40]

Clinical guidance
Absorption may be reduced if administered via jejunostomy, although this is not believed to be a problem.[158] Monitor effect and consider checking drug levels if necessary. The elixir has a high osmolality.

Malabsorption has occurred in patients with small intestine disease or short bowel syndrome.[155]

The elixir has a different bioavailability from the tablets so dose adjustments may be necessary.[90] However this is controversial as the manufacturers of Lanoxin PG® say that no dosage adjustment is necessary when switching from tablets to elixir. Contact Pharmacy for advice.

62.5mcg tablet	equivalent to	50mcg (1ml) elixir

Feed guidance
The absorption of digoxin is affected by high fibre feeds such as Jevity®. Allow a time gap of two hours before and two hours after administration of digoxin before administering high fibre enteral feeds.

Dihydrocodeine

Presentation
Tablets.
Suspension.
Modified-release tablets.

Administration - enteral tubes / swallowing difficulties
Use the suspension.[41] Follow the directions in section 3.6.

Do not crush the modified-release tablets. Contact Pharmacy for advice.

Di-iodohydroxyquinoline

Presentation
Tablets (named patient).

Administration – enteral tubes
No information about the use of this medication via enteral feeding tubes has been located.

Administration – swallowing difficulties
The tablets can be crushed and mixed with apple sauce or chocolate syrup for patients with swallowing difficulties.[152]

Diloxanide

Presentation
Tablets.

Administration – enteral tubes
No information about the use of this medication via enteral feeding tubes has been located.

Administration – swallowing difficulties
The tablets can be crushed and mixed with water for administration.[152]

Diltiazem

Presentation
Modified-release tablets, modified-release capsules.

Administration – enteral tubes
All tablets and capsules are labelled as modified-release, however the 60mg generic preparation is not slow release and can be crushed.[14] Contact Pharmacy for advice if unsure. Follow the directions in section 3.5. Contact Pharmacy for advice on equivalent doses. A suspension may be prepared by Pharmacy in some centres.[155]

Viazem® XL and Adizem® MR capsules have been opened for administration via wide bore enteral feeding tubes.[132] The capsule contents should not be crushed.

Administration – swallowing difficulties
The MR capsules have been opened and the contents mixed with soft food for administration. Do not crush the capsule contents.[132] This method may not be suitable for patients with limited understanding or impaired ability to follow instructions.

Alternatively, switch to amlodipine. Contact Pharmacy for advice.

Dinoprostone

Presentation
Tablets.
Injection.

Administration - enteral tubes / swallowing difficulties
The injection can be diluted with water for use enterally.[40,160] Follow the directions in section 3.6.

Dipyridamole

Presentation
Sugar-coated tablets.
Modified-release capsules.
Injection.
Suspension.

Administration – enteral tubes
1st choice – Use the suspension. Follow the directions in section 3.6.
2nd choice – Use the injection enterally.[44,152] Follow the directions in section 3.6.

Administration – swallowing difficulties
1st choice – Use the suspension.

The modified-release capsule contents have been mixed with soft food for administration to patients with swallowing difficulties, but this is not recommended. The capsule contents should not be crushed, therefore this method may not be suitable with limited understanding or impaired ability to follow instructions.[132]

Clinical guidance
A dosage adjustment is required when switching from modified-release capsules to suspension. Contact Pharmacy for advice.

Feed guidance
Dipyridamole should be given on an empty stomach, so withhold enteral feeds for one hour before and one hour after dose.[117]

Disodium etidronate

Presentation
Tablets.

Administration - enteral tubes / swallowing difficulties
1st choice – A suspension can be prepared by Pharmacy in some centres. Follow the directions in section 3.6.
2nd choice – The tablet can be crushed and dispersed in water for administration via enteral feeding tube.[104,105] Follow the directions in section 3.5. If giving via enteral feeding tube, flush post dose with 50ml of distilled water.

Feed guidance
Stop feed two hours before and two hours after administration of etidronate.

Disopyramide

Presentation
Capsules.
Modified-release tablets.
Injection.

Administration - enteral tubes / swallowing difficulties
1st choice – The standard capsules can be opened and the contents mixed with water for administration.[87] Follow the directions in section 3.7.
2nd choice – The injection can be used enterally if necessary. It has a strong, bitter taste, and a local anaesthetic effect in the mouth, and so should be used with care if given orally to patients with swallowing difficulties.[40,97] Follow the directions in section 3.6.

The modified-release tablets should not be used. Contact Pharmacy for advice for patients maintained on modified-release tablets.

Docusate

Presentation
Capsules.
Oral solution, paediatric oral suspension.

Administration - enteral tubes / swallowing difficulties
Use the oral solution. Follow the directions in section 3.6. Do not open the capsules.[41]

Domperidone

Presentation
Tablets.
Sugar-free suspension.
Suppositories.

Administration - enteral tubes
1st choice – Use the suppositories if possible (contact Pharmacy for advice on dose conversion).
2nd choice – Use the suspension (contains sorbitol[104]) and dilute with an equal amount of water before administration.[133] Follow the directions in section 3.6.

Administration - swallowing difficulties
Use the suppositories (contact Pharmacy for advice on dose conversion) or the suspension (contains sorbitol[104]).

Donepezil

Presentation
Film-coated tablets.

Administration - enteral tubes / swallowing difficulties
The tablets can be crushed and mixed with water for administration.[104,105] Follow the directions in section 3.5. Has a strong, bitter taste.[150]

Dosulepin (Dothiepin)

Presentation
Tablets, capsules.
Sugar-free oral solution (special).

Administration - enteral tubes / swallowing difficulties
Use the oral solution.[104] Follow the directions in section 3.6.

The tablets have been crushed and the capsules have been opened, but this is not recommended as the tablets are very hard[132] and the powder has a local anaesthetic action.[105]

Doxazosin

Presentation
Tablets.
Modified-release tablets.

Administration - enteral tubes / swallowing difficulties
The standard tablets disperse readily in deionised water for administration.[37] Most disperse within one minute.[154] Do not use tap water, as the chloride ions in the water will cause the drug to precipitate out.[104,105] Use deionised water for flushing enteral feeding tubes following each dose. Follow the directions in section 3.5.

The modified-release tablets are not suitable for enteral tube administration and should not be crushed. A dose adjustment and blood pressure monitoring may be necessary when switching from modified-release tablets to standard tablets. Contact Pharmacy for advice.

Deionised water must be used, and no other drugs / fluids should be mixed with doxazosin as the drug will precipitate in the presence of chloride ions. Flush enteral feeding tubes well with water before and after each dose.[37]

Doxepin

Presentation
Capsules.

Administration - enteral tubes / swallowing difficulties
The capsules can be opened, and the contents dispersed in water.[37]
Follow the directions in section 3.7. The powder has a bitter taste.[105]

Doxycycline

Presentation
Capsules.
Dispersible tablets.

Administration - enteral tubes / swallowing difficulties
Use the dispersible tablets. Follow the directions in section 3.5.
Do not open the capsules as the contents are irritant.[94]

Clinical guidance
Doxycycline binds to calcium ions and may have reduced absorption
when given via enteral feeding tubes. Prescribe at the higher end of
the standard dosage range.[94]

Feed guidance
Withhold enteral feeds for one hour before and two hours after each
dose.[117]

Dydrogesterone

Presentation
Tablets.

Administration - enteral tubes / swallowing difficulties
The tablets can be crushed (preferably in water to reduce dust
production) and mixed with water for administration.[105] Follow the
directions in section 3.5.

Efavirenz

Presentation
Film-coated tablets, capsules.
Oral solution.

Administration - enteral tubes / swallowing difficulties
Use the oral solution and dilute with water before administration.[132]
Follow the directions in section 3.6.

Clinical guidance
A dose conversion is necessary when switching from tablets to solution. Contact Pharmacy for advice.

600mg tablet	equivalent to	720mg solution[132]

Emtricitabine

Presentation
Capsules.

Administration - enteral tubes / swallowing difficulties
The capsules can be opened and the contents dispersed in water for administration.[132] Follow the directions in section 3.7.

Enalapril

Presentation
Tablets.
A suspension can be made by Pharmacy.[150]

Administration - enteral tubes / swallowing difficulties
1st choice – Use the suspension if available.
2nd choice – The tablets can be crushed and dispersed in water for administration.[40,41,152] Without crushing they disperse in around five minutes.[154] Follow the directions in section 3.5. The crushed tablets may have a bitter after-taste.[135]

Entacapone

Presentation
Film-coated tablets.

Administration – enteral tubes
The tablets can be dispersed in water for administration.[104,105] They disperse in one to five minutes.[154] Follow the directions in section 3.5. Take care if crushing as this produces red dust which may stain.[132]

Entacapone does not fully dissolve in water, so if giving via enteral feeding tube, flush well after administration. The drug also stains orange, and may stain an enteral feeding tube.[105]

Administration – swallowing difficulties
The crushed tablet may be given in jam, honey, or orange juice as it has a bitter taste.[104,132]

Eprosartan

Presentation
Film-coated tablets.

Administration - enteral tubes / swallowing difficulties
The tablets can be crushed and mixed with water for administration.[138] Follow the directions in section 3.5.

Erythromycin

Presentation
Capsules.
Film-coated tablets.
Suspension.
Injection.

Administration - enteral tubes / swallowing difficulties
1st choice – Give by parenteral injection.
2nd choice – Use the suspension.[94,104] Follow the directions in section 3.6.

Escitalopram

Presentation
Film-coated tablets.

Administration - enteral tubes
1st choice – Consider switching to citalopram as this is available in a liquid form. Contact Pharmacy for advice on citalopram dosage.
2nd choice – The tablets can be dispersed in water for administration.[105] They disperse immediately.[154] Follow the directions in section 3.5. Flush well as the tablets are poorly soluble.[132]

Administration - swallowing difficulties
1st choice – Consider switching to citalopram as this is available in a liquid form. Contact Pharmacy for advice on citalopram dosage.
2nd choice – The tablets can be dispersed in water for administration.[105] They disperse immediately.[154] Follow the directions in section 3.5. The crushed / dispersed tablets have an unpleasant taste.[132]

Esomeprazole

Presentation
Film-coated tablets.

Administration - enteral tubes
Esomeprazole tablets are licensed for administration via gastric tubes.[156] They will disperse in water for administration. The pellets remaining after the tablet disperses should not be crushed.[156]

1. Place the tablet in the barrel of an oral or bladder-tipped syringe.
2. Draw up 25ml water and 5ml air.
3. Shake the syringe for 2 minutes to disperse the tablet.
4. Hold the tip upright to ensure it has not clogged with particles.
5. Attach to the tube whilst keeping the tip upright.
6. Shake the syringe, point it down, and administer 5-10ml of the contents.
7. Invert the syringe and shake.
8. Point the tip down and administer another 5-10ml.
9. Repeat until empty.
10. Draw up another 25ml of water and 5ml of air, and administer to wash the sediment from syringe.[156]

This is only suitable for fairly wide bore tubes. The 20mg tablets can be administered through tubes size 8 French and larger, the 40mg through 14 French and larger.[132] Follow the directions in section 3.5.

Administration - swallowing difficulties
The tablets can be dispersed in water for administration. The pellets remaining after the tablet disperses should not be crushed.[156]

1. Place the tablet in the barrel of an oral or bladder-tipped syringe.
2. Draw up 25ml water and 5ml air.
3. Shake the syringe for 2 minutes to disperse the tablet.
4. Hold the tip upright to ensure it has not clogged with particles.
5. Shake the syringe, point it down, and administer 5-10ml to the patient.
6. Invert the syringe and shake.
7. Point the tip down and administer another 5-10ml.
8. Repeat until empty.
9. Draw up another 25ml of water and 5ml of air, and administer to wash the sediment from syringe.[156]

Etamsylate (Ethamsylate)

Presentation
Tablets.

Administration - enteral tubes / swallowing difficulties
The tablets can be crushed and mixed with water for
administration.[104] Follow the directions in section 3.5.

Ethambutol

Presentation
Tablets.

Administration - enteral tubes / swallowing difficulties
1st choice – A liquid can be prepared by Pharmacy in some
centres.[95] Follow the directions in section 3.6.
2nd choice – The tablets can be crushed and mixed with water for
administration.[104,105] Follow the directions in section 3.5.

Ethosuximide

Presentation
Capsules.
Syrup.

Administration - enteral tubes / swallowing difficulties
Use the syrup.[41,104] Follow the directions in section 3.6.

Etoposide

Presentation
Capsules.
Injection.

Administration - enteral tubes / swallowing difficulties
<u>Caution – cytotoxic.</u> Contact Pharmacy for advice before giving.
The injection has been diluted to 0.4mg/ml with water for
administration via enteral feeding tubes, or in orange juice for oral
administration in some centres.[138]

Ezetimibe

Presentation
Tablets.

Clinical Guidance
Not suitable for administration via enteral feeding tubes as the
excipients do not mix well with water. There is no data on drug
stability or whether the drug may interact with enteral feeding
tubes.[124]

Famciclovir

Presentation
Tablets.

Administration - enteral tubes / swallowing difficulties
The tablets can be crushed and mixed with water for
administration.[105] Follow the directions in section 3.5.

Famotidine

Presentation
Tablets.

Administration - enteral tubes / swallowing difficulties
The tablets can be crushed and mixed with water for administration.[134] Follow the directions in section 3.5.

Felodipine

Clinical guidance
Felodipine tablets should not be crushed and are not suitable for enteral feeding tube administration.[60] Consider amlodipine as an alternative. Contact Pharmacy for advice.

Fenofibrate

Presentation
Capsules.
Modified-release tablets.

Administration – enteral tubes
The capsules can be opened and the contents dispersed in water.[61] Follow the directions in section 3.7.

Administration – swallowing difficulties
The capsule contents have also been administered in orange juice to patients with swallowing difficulties.[105]

The modified-release tablet is not suitable for crushing. Contact Pharmacy for advice.

Ferrous sulphate

Clinical guidance
See entry under 'Iron preparations'

Fexofenadine

Presentation
Film-coated tablets.

Administration - enteral tubes / swallowing difficulties
1st choice – Switch to an alternative antihistamine available as a liquid, e.g. loratadine.
2nd choice – The tablets can be crushed and mixed with water for adminstration.[62] Without crushing they disperse in around five minutes.[154] Follow the directions in section 3.5.

Feed guidance
Tablets should be given on an empty stomach, so withhold enteral feeds for two hours before and two hours after administration.[62]

Finasteride

Presentation
Film-coated tablets.

Administration - enteral tubes / swallowing difficulties
Place the tablet in the barrel of an oral or bladder-tipped syringe. Draw water up into the syringe and allow the tablet to disperse[63] (in order to minimise contact). Follow the directions in section 3.5. If giving via enteral feeding tube, flush well after each dose as the drug is insoluble.[155]

Women who are or who may become pregnant should not handle crushed, broken, or dissolved tablets.[64]

Flavoxate

Presentation
Film-coated tablets.

Administration - enteral tubes
The tablets can be crushed and mixed with water for administration.[105] Follow the directions in section 3.5. Flush enteral tubes well after dosing.[105]

Administration - swallowing difficulties
The tablets can be crushed and mixed with water for administration.[105] Follow the directions in section 3.5. Flavoxate has a bitter taste when crushed.[105]

Flecainide

Presentation
Tablets.
Oral liquid (contains sorbitol).
Injection.

Administration - enteral tubes / swallowing difficulties
1st choice – Use the liquid. Follow the directions in section 3.6.
2nd choice – The tablets can be crushed and dispersed in deionised water for administration.[40] Some sources do not recommend this.[152] Follow the directions in section 3.5. Do not use tap water.[105] The crushed tablets have a local anaesthetic effect, so should be used with care in patients with swallowing difficulties.[40]
3rd choice – The injection has been administered enterally, given undiluted. This should only be used in emergency situations, and the patient should be monitored for clinical / adverse effects.[40,168] Follow the directions in section 3.6.

Clinical guidance
If giving via enteral feeding tube, always flush with deionised water, and do not mix with alkali solutions, sulphate, phosphate, or chloride ions.[95] Do NOT mix this drug with other medications prior to administration.

Flucloxacillin

Presentation
Capsules.
Suspension.
Injection.

Administration - enteral tubes / swallowing difficulties
1st choice – Give by parenteral injection.
2nd choice – Use the suspension. Follow the directions in section 3.6.

Clinical guidance
The suspension has a high osmolality. Administer reconstituted injection via the enteral feeding tube in patients with tubes delivering directly into the jejunum if osmotic diarrhoea is a problem.[104,155] It is likely that flucloxacillin has a similar absorption following administration directly into the jejunum as it does following oral administration.[158]

Feed guidance
Stop enteral feeds for one hour before and one-two hours after administration of flucloxacillin suspension.[104] Flucloxacillin has to be given on an empty stomach.[35] If this is not possible then consider increasing the dose and decreasing the frequency of administration.

Fluconazole

Presentation
Capsules.
Suspension.
Infusion.

Administration - enteral tubes / swallowing difficulties
1st choice – Give by intravenous infusion if appropriate.
2nd choice – Use the suspension.[104] Follow the directions in section 3.6.
3rd choice – The capsules can be opened, and the contents mixed with water for administration.[155] Follow the directions in section 3.7.

Clinical guidance
Higher doses may be required when administered directly into the jejunum.[155]

Feed guidance
Fluconazole interacts with Jevity® enteral feeds. Stop enteral feeds for one hour before and one hour after each dose of fluconazole.[105]

Fludrocortisone

Presentation
Tablets.

Administration - enteral tubes / swallowing difficulties
1st choice – A suspension can be made by Pharmacy at some centres. Follow the directions in section 3.6.
2nd choice – The tablets will disperse in water.[7,40,41,152] They disperse within one minute.[154] Follow the directions in section 3.5. If giving via enteral feeding tube, flush well after administration.[155]

Fluoxetine

Presentation
Capsules.
Liquid.

Administration - enteral tubes / swallowing difficulties
1st choice – Use the liquid (and if giving via enteral feeding tube, dilute with the same volume of distilled water). Follow the directions in section 3.6.
2nd choice – The capsules have been opened and the contents dispersed in 120ml water. The capsule contents will dissolve in about 5 minutes.[132] Follow the directions in section 3.7.

Clinical guidance
Absorption of fluoxetine appears to occur through the gastrointestinal tract [9,16] and it is well absorbed when given through enteral tubes terminating in the jejunum. Fluoxetine liquid does not contain sorbitol.

Flupentixol (Flupenthixol)

Presentation
Sugar-coated tablets.
Depot injections.

Administration – enteral tubes
The tablets can be crushed and mixed with water for administration.[105] Follow the directions in section 3.5. The tablets are poorly soluble, so flush well after dosing.

Administration – swallowing difficulties
Crushed tablets can also be mixed with fruit juice for administration to patients with swallowing difficulties.[104] Give immediately after mixing with fruit juice.[104]

Fluphenazine

Presentation
Sugar-coated tablets.

Administration - enteral tubes / swallowing difficulties
The tablets can be crushed and dispersed in water for administration (some centres advise against this).[41,95] Follow the directions in section 3.5.

Flurbiprofen

Presentation
Tablets, sugar-coated tablets.
Modified-release capsules.

Administration - enteral tubes / swallowing difficulties
The capsules can be opened and the modified-release microbeads administered in plenty of water. The onset of action may be faster when the drug is administered in this way. The microbeads should not be crushed, and may have the potential to block narrow bore enteral feeding tubes.[138] Follow the directions in section 3.7.

Flutamide

Presentation
Tablets.

Administration - enteral tubes / swallowing difficulties
The tablets can be crushed and mixed with milk or fruit juice for administration.[105] Follow the directions in section 3.5.

Fluvastatin

Presentation
Capsules.
Modified-release tablets.

Administration - enteral tubes / swallowing difficulties
The capsules can be opened and the contents mixed with water for administration.[41,65] Follow the directions in section 3.7. There is no information available on whether fluvastatin is likely to block enteral feeding tubes. When giving via enteral tube, flush well after each dose.[65]

The modified-release tablet is not suitable for tube administration. Contact Pharmacy for advice.

Fluvoxamine

Presentation
Tablets.
Film-coated tablets.

Administration - enteral tubes / swallowing difficulties
The tablets can be crushed and mixed with water for administration.[105] Follow the directions in section 3.5.

Folic acid

Presentation
Tablets.
Syrup.
Injection (unlicensed special).

Administration - enteral tubes / swallowing difficulties
1st choice – Use the syrup.[94,104] Follow the directions in section 3.6.
2nd choice – The tablets have been crushed and mixed with water for administration.[133] Follow the directions in section 3.5.

Forceval

Presentation
Capsules and junior capsules.

Administration - enteral tubes / swallowing difficulties
1st choice – Consider switching to an alternate multivitamin preparation available as a liquid. Contact Pharmacy for advice.
2nd choice – Snip off the end of the forceval capsule and withdraw the contents using a syringe. – Take great care when using a syringe to prepare an ORAL / ENTERAL dosage. The contents of forceval capsules taste foul, and do not mix well with water.[132] This method is not recommended.

Fosinopril

Presentation
Tablets.

Administration - enteral tubes / swallowing difficulties
The tablets can be crushed and mixed with water for administration.[105] Follow the directions in section 3.5.

Furazolidone

Presentation
Tablets (named patient).
Oral suspension (named patient).

Administration – enteral tubes
No information about the use of this medication via enteral feeding tubes has been located.

Administration – swallowing difficulties
The tablets can be crushed and mixed with a spoonful of corn syrup.[152,157]

Furosemide (Frusemide)

Presentation
Tablets.
Sugar-free oral solution (some preparations contain alcohol).
Injection.

Administration - enteral tubes / swallowing difficulties
1st choice – Consider giving by parenteral injection.
2nd choice – Use the oral solution (and when giving via enteral feeding tube, dilute with the same volume of water).[94] Follow the directions in section 3.6.

Clinical guidance
Absorption may be reduced when administered directly into the jejunum.[104,158]

Gabapentin

Presentation
Tablets, capsules.
Syrup (imported special – Pfizer[145])

Administration – enteral tubes
Open the capsule, dissolve the contents in water, and give immediately (gabapentin has limited stability in water).[37,41,152] Follow the directions in section 3.7.

Administration – swallowing difficulties
The contents of the capsules can be sprinkled on food or given in fruit juice to mask their unpleasant taste. They should be given immediately as the drug is rapidly hydrolysed.[37,104]

Clinical guidance
Do not give at the same time as aluminium / magnesium antacids.[35]

Galantamine

Presentation
Film-coated tablets.
Modified-release capsules.
Solution.

Administration - enteral tubes / swallowing difficulties
1st choice – Use the solution if it is available. Follow the directions in section 3.6.
2nd choice – The tablets can be crushed and mixed with water for administration.[104] Follow the directions in section 3.5.

Ganciclovir

Presentation
Capsules.
Infusion.

Clinical guidance
Ganciclovir is toxic. Do not open the capsule.[41] Contact Pharmacy for advice.

Glibenclamide

Presentation
Tablets.

Administration - enteral tubes / swallowing difficulties
1st choice – Consider whether switching to insulin would be appropriate.
2nd choice – A suspension may be available from Pharmacy at some centres.[155] Follow the directions in section 3.6.
3rd choice – The tablets can be crushed and mixed with water for administration.[62] Without crushing they disperse in around five minutes.[154] Follow the directions in section 3.5.

Clinical guidance
There is a possibility of reduced absorption when administered directly into the jejunum.[155]

Feed guidance
Give just before the start of a feed.[62]

Gliclazide

Presentation
Tablets.
Modified-release tablets.

Administration - enteral tubes / swallowing difficulties
1st choice – Consider whether switching to insulin would be appropriate.
2nd choice – A suspension may be available from Pharmacy at some centres.[155] Follow the directions in section 3.6.
3rd choice – Crush the tablets well and mix with water or orange juice for administration.[45,132] Follow the directions in section 3.5.

Do not crush the modified-release tablets.

Feed guidance
Give just before the start of a feed.[132]

Glimepiride

Presentation
Tablets.

Clinical guidance
Do not crush the tablets as this may affect their bioavailability.[62]
Consider whether switching to insulin would be appropriate.

Glipizide

Presentation
Tablets.

Administration - enteral tubes / swallowing difficulties
1st choice – Consider whether switching to insulin would be appropriate.
2nd choice – The tablets can be crushed and dispersed in water for administration.[66] Follow the directions in section 3.5. There is no information available on whether glipizide is likely to block enteral feeding tubes.[66]

Gliquidone

Presentation
Tablets.

Administration - enteral tubes / swallowing difficulties
1st choice – Consider whether switching to insulin would be appropriate.
2nd choice – The tablets can be crushed and dispersed in water for administration.[138] Follow the directions in section 3.5.

Glyceryl trinitrate

Presentation
Acute use preparations.
Sublingual tablets.
Sublingual spray.
Injection.

Prophylaxis preparations.
Modified-release buccal tablets.
Modified-release tablets.
Transdermal patches.
Ointment.

Administration - enteral tubes / swallowing difficulties
Acute use preparations.
For patients with an unsafe swallow, use the sublingual spray.

Prophylaxis preparations.
Buccal tablets can be continued in patients who are able to use them
appropriately.

Do not crush the modified release tablets. Consider switching
patients on modified-release tablets intended for swallowing to
transdermal patches. Contact Pharmacy for advice.

Clinical guidance
The sublingual and buccal tablets require moisture in the mouth for
adequate absorption, and may be less effective in patients with
swallowing difficulties.

Glycopyrronium

Presentation
Tablets (named patient only).[40]
Injection.

Administration - enteral tubes / swallowing difficulties
1st choice – Consider using subcutaneous doses when required, or a subcutaneous infusion by syringe driver.
2nd choice – If the tablets are available, they can be crushed and mixed with water for administration.[40,152] Follow the directions in section 3.5.
3rd choice – The injection has been used orally and via enteral feeding tubes.[132,152] Follow the directions in section 3.6.

Granisetron

Presentation
Film-coated tablets.
Liquid.
Injection.

Administration - enteral tubes / swallowing difficulties
1st choice – Give by parenteral injection.
2nd choice – Use the liquid, and flush with 15-30ml of distilled water.[41] Follow the directions in section 3.6.

Haloperidol

Presentation
Tablets, capsules.
Oral liquid.
Injection, depot injection.

Administration - enteral tubes / swallowing difficulties
1st choice – Give by parenteral injection if appropriate.
2nd choice – Use the liquid preparation (and when giving via enteral feeding tube, dilute with the same volume of distilled water). Follow the directions in section 3.6.
3rd choice – The capsules can be opened and the contents dispersed in water.[133] Follow the directions in section 3.7.

Hydralazine

Presentation
Sugar-coated tablets.
Injection.

Administration - enteral tubes / swallowing difficulties
1st choice – A suspension may be available from Pharmacy at some centres.[155] Follow the directions in section 3.6.
2nd choice - The injection can be made up with water for injections and administered orally or via enteral feeding tubes.[40,98,152] Follow the directions in section 3.6.
3rd choice – The tablets can be crushed,[98] but are sugar-coated and are likely to block enteral feeding tubes. Follow the directions in section 3.5.

Clinical guidance
Hydralazine absorption is reduced in the presence of enteral feeds. Withhold the feed for two hours before and one hour after each dose.[155] Crushing the tablets may also alter their absorption rate (usually increased).[105] Monitor blood pressure.[87,90,95]

Hydralazine injection, when used for oral / enteral feeding tube administration, should only be made up with water for injections, as it interacts with metal ions found in other water sources.[98]

Hydrocortisone

Presentation
Tablets.
Injection.

Administration - enteral tubes / swallowing difficulties
1st choice – Give by parenteral injection if possible.
2nd choice – A suspension can be made by Pharmacy in some centres.[63] Follow the directions in section 3.6.
3rd choice – The tablets are insoluble but will disperse in water for administration.[63,152] They disperse within one minute.[154] Follow the directions in section 3.5.
4th choice – Efcortesol® injection may be given enterally.[152] Follow the directions in section 3.6.

Hydromorphone

Presentation
Capsules.
Modified-release capsules.

Clinical Guidance
Not recommended as there is a high incidence of tube blockage.[149]
Contact Pharmacy for advice.

Hydroxycarbamide (Hydroxyurea)

Presentation
Capsules.

Administration - enteral tubes / swallowing difficulties
Caution – cytotoxic. Contact Pharmacy for advice before giving. The capsules are cytotoxic and should not be opened except on Pharmacy advice. If no other method is appropriate, on advice from Pharmacy the capsules can be opened and the contents dispersed in water for administration.[105] Follow the directions in section 3.7.

Hydroxychloroquine

Presentation
Film-coated tablets.

Administration - enteral tubes / swallowing difficulties
1st choice – A liquid can be prepared by Pharmacy at some centres.[95] Follow the directions in section 3.6.
2nd choice – The tablets can be crushed and dispersed in water for administration.[104,105,152] Follow the directions in section 3.5.

Hydroxyzine

Presentation
Sugar-coated tablets.
Syrup.

Administration - enteral tubes / swallowing difficulties
Use the syrup.[94,104] Follow the directions in section 3.6.

Hyoscine butylbromide

Presentation
Coated tablets.
Injection.

Administration - enteral tubes / swallowing difficulties
Do not crush the tablet. The injection can be administered enterally.[40,44,152] Follow the directions in section 3.6.

Hyoscine hydrobromide

Presentation
Tablets.
Transdermal patch (Scopoderm).
Injection.

Administration - enteral tubes / swallowing difficulties
1st choice – Consider using the patch or giving by parenteral injection.
2nd choice – The tablets may be sucked if the patient is able, and absorbed through the lining of the mouth,[103] although the level of absorption may vary, particularly in patients with little saliva.
3rd choice – The tablets can be dissolved[103] in water for administration via enteral tube, but again, absorption may vary. Follow the directions in section 3.5.
4th choice – The injection has been used enterally.[138,160] Follow the directions in section 3.6.

Ibuprofen

Presentation
Sugar-coated tablets.
Syrup, effervescent sachets.
Modified-release tablets, modified-release capsules.

Administration - enteral tubes / swallowing difficulties
1st choice – Consider using an alternative non-steroidal anti-inflammatory drug available as injection or suppositories, e.g. diclofenac.
2nd choice – Use the syrup.[104] Follow the directions in section 3.6.

Imipramine

Presentation
Coated tablets.
Syrup (may not be available).

Administration - enteral tubes
1st choice – Use the syrup, if available.[104,105] Follow the directions in section 3.6. The drug may adsorb to the tube, so flush well after dosing.
2nd choice – The tablets may be crushed and mixed with water for administration. Flush well after dosing as the coating has the potential to block enteral feeding tubes.[133] Follow the directions in section 3.5.

Administration - swallowing difficulties
1st choice – Use the syrup, if available.[104,105] Follow the directions in section 3.6.
2nd choice – The tablets may be crushed and mixed with water for administration.[133] Follow the directions in section 3.5.

Indapamide

Presentation
Coated tablets.
Modified-release tablets.

Administration – NG / PEG tubes / swallowing difficulties
For patients with tubes terminating in the stomach, the standard tablets can be dispersed in water for administration.[104,105] They disperse in one to five minutes.[154] Follow the directions in section 3.5.

Do not crush the modified-release tablets.

Administration – NJ / PEJ / PEGJ tubes
Administration via tubes terminating in the jejunum is not appropriate for indapamide as absorption will be greatly reduced. Contact Pharmacy for advice.[155]

Indometacin (Indomethacin)

Presentation
Capsules.
Sugar-free suspension.
Suppositories.
Modified-release tablets, modified-release capsules.

Administration - enteral tubes / swallowing difficulties
1st choice – Use the suppositories if possible.
2nd choice – Use the suspension. Follow the directions in section 3.6.

The modified-release capsules are irritant to the stomach, and should not be opened.

Do not crush the tablets.

Indoramin

Presentation
Tablets.

Administration – enteral tubes
The tablets can be dispersed in water for administration.[67] They disperse immediately.[154] Protect from light.[138] Follow the directions in section 3.5.

Administration – swallowing difficulties
The tablets can be crushed and sprinkled onto soft food to mask the taste.[105]

Inositol nicotinate

Presentation
Tablets.

Administration – enteral tubes
No information about the use of this medication via enteral feeding tubes has been located.

Administration – swallowing difficulties
The tablets will not dissolve but can be crushed and mixed with soft food for patients with swallowing difficulties.[132]

Irbesartan

Presentation
Tablets.

Administration - enteral tubes / swallowing difficulties
Tablets can be crushed and dispersed in water for administration.[68] Without crushing they disperse in around five minutes.[154] Follow the directions in section 3.5. There is no information available to indicate whether irbesartan is likely to block enteral feeding tubes.[68] When giving via enteral feeding tube, flush well after each dose as the drug is practically insoluble.[155]

Iron preparations

Presentation
Various.

Administration - enteral tubes / swallowing difficulties
Use ferrous fumarate liquid. Follow the directions in section 3.6.

When administering via enteral tubes terminating in the jejunum, absorption may be decreased.[155]

Preparations[35]

Ferrous sulphate 200mg tablets contain 65mg of iron	Ferrous fumarate 140mg/5ml syrup contains 45mg/5ml of iron

Equivalent doses

200mg FeSO4 tablet 200mg three times daily	equivalent to equivalent to	7.2ml ferrous fumarate syrup 10ml twice daily

Isoniazid

Presentation
Tablets.
Oral solution (special).
Injection.

Administration - enteral tubes / swallowing difficulties
1st choice – Use the oral solution if it is available.[104] Follow the directions in section 3.6.
2nd choice – The tablets can be crushed and mixed with water for administration.[105] Follow the directions in section 3.5.

Feed guidance
Isoniazid should be given on an empty stomach. Hold enteral feeds for one hour before and one hour after dose.[117]

Isosorbide dinitrate

Presentation
Tablets.
Modified-release tablets.

Administration - enteral tubes / swallowing difficulties
The standard release tablets can be crushed and will disperse in water with a fine sediment.[7,40,94] Follow the directions in section 3.5.

There is a theoretical potential for explosion if isosorbide dinitrate tablets are crushed. However no reports of this occurring have been located, and the practice is carried out in many centres.

Do not crush the modified-release tablets. Contact Pharmacy for advice.

Isosorbide mononitrate

Presentation
Tablets.
Modified-release tablets, modified-release capsules.

Administration - enteral tubes / swallowing difficulties
1st choice – A suspension can be made by Pharmacy in some centres. Follow the directions in section 3.6.
2nd choice – The standard release tablets can be crushed and dispersed in water.[39,40,41] They may have an increased rate of absorption and therefore increased side effects.[104] Follow the directions in section 3.5.

Do not crush the modified-release tablets.

There is a theoretical potential for explosion if isosorbide mononitrate tablets are crushed. However no reports of this occurring have been located, and the practice is carried out in many centres. The manufacturers do not believe there to be any risk.[159]

Clinical guidance
Modified-release tablets and capsules are not suitable for enteral feeding tube administration. Contact Pharmacy for advice on adjusting doses and switching preparations. Alternatively, consider using GTN patches.

Feed guidance
The modified-release capsules may be opened and the contents mixed with soft food for administration to patients with swallowing difficulties, but this is not recommended. Do not crush the capsule contents or pre-dissolve them before giving.[132,155]

Isotretinoin

Presentation
Capsules.

Administration - enteral tubes / swallowing difficulties
Caution – teratogenic. Special precautions are required in certain female patients during the use of this drug. Contact Pharmacy for advice.

Use a needle and a 1ml oral syringe to pierce the capsule and withdraw the fluid contents (squeeze the capsule at the same time to aid withdrawal). Flush the fluid down the enteral feeding tube with water, or mix with food for oral administration.[138]

Give immediately. Be aware that serious errors have occurred due to the use of needles and syringes to handle oral medication.

Ispaghula husk

Clinical Guidance
Do not use as it may congeal and block the tube.

Isradipine

Presentation
Tablets.

Administration - enteral tubes / swallowing difficulties
The tablets can be crushed and dispersed in water for administration. Protect from light.[138] Follow the directions in section 3.5.

Itraconazole

Presentation
Capsules.
Liquid.
Concentrate for infusion.

Administration - enteral tubes / swallowing difficulties
1st choice – Give by parenteral infusion if appropriate.
2nd choice – Use the liquid.[104] Follow the directions in section 3.6.

Use of the capsule contents has led to enteral feeding tube blockage, so this is not recommended.[138]

Feed guidance
Itraconazole should be given on an empty stomach so withhold enteral feeds for one hour before each dose.[41]

Ketoconazole

Presentation
Tablets.

Administration – NG / PEG tubes / swallowing difficulties
1st choice – A suspension may be available from Pharmacy at some centres.[155] Follow the directions in section 3.6.
2nd choice - The tablets can be crushed and dispersed in water for administration.[104,105] Follow the directions in section 3.5.

Administration – NJ / PEJ / PEGJ tubes
Administration of ketoconazole directly into the jejunum is not recommended as a low pH is required for absorption of this drug.[104,158]

Clinical guidance
Do not give antacids at the same time as this medication.[155]

Labetalol

Presentation
Tablets.
Injection.

Administration – enteral tubes
The injection can be given via enteral feeding tube.[40,99,152] Follow the directions in section 3.6.

Administration – swallowing difficulties
Mix the required dose of injection with orange juice to disguise the bitter taste.[40,99,152] The tablets have been crushed but the powder tastes unpleasant,[105] and this is not recommended because the drug is sensitive to oxidation.[132]

Lacidipine

Presentation
Tablets.

Clinical guidance
The tablets are very insoluble and film coated, and are likely to block enteral feeding tubes.[44] They have been crushed but this is not recommended.[132] Contact Pharmacy for advice.

Lactulose

Presentation
Solution.

Administration - enteral tubes / swallowing difficulties
Dilute solution 1 in 3 or 1 in 4 with distilled water (i.e. dilute each 10ml with 30ml water).

Lactulose is almost completely unabsorbed in the GI tract.[1] It acts by local action in the colon and is therefore equally effective when given through a tube terminating in the jejunum as when given orally.

Lamivudine

Presentation
Film-coated tablets.
Oral solution.

Administration - enteral tubes / swallowing difficulties
Use the oral solution.[132] Follow the directions in section 3.6.

Lamotrigine

Presentation
Tablets.
Dispersible tablets.

Administration - enteral tubes / swallowing difficulties
Use the dispersible tablets. Follow the directions in section 3.5.

Lansoprazole

Presentation
Capsules.
"FasTabs".
Suspension in sachet form.

Administration – enteral tubes
1. Place the 'Fastab' tablet in the barrel of an oral or bladder-tipped syringe, then draw up 10-20ml water.
2. Shake and allow the tablet to disperse.
3. Administer the solution via the enteral tube with repeated shaking to suspend the microgranules. Do not crush the microgranules as the syringe empties.
4. Draw up another 10ml water and repeat the process until all the granules have been administered.
5. Flush the tube well following administration.

For patients with tubes terminating in the jejunum, some sources recommend adding the contents of the capsule to 10ml of sodium bicarbonate 8.4% in an oral or bladder-tipped syringe.[155] Any resulting gas should be allowed to escape.

Lansoprazole suspension (sachets) interacts with enteral feeding tubes and is therefore unsuitable for use except in patients with swallowing difficulties.

Administration – swallowing difficulties
The "FasTab" will disperse in water, leaving microgranules, which should not be crushed, or can be administered in apple juice or orange juice.[105] Alternatively, use the sachets.

Feed guidance
Lansoprazole should be given on an empty stomach, so withhold enteral feeds for one hour before and one hour after each dose.[117]

Leflunomide

Presentation
Tablets.

Clinical guidance
There is no information available on the use of leflunomide via enteral feeding tubes, however there is no pharmaceutical reason why the tablets shouldn't be crushed, and this has been done in some centres. If administering crushed tablets, monitor the patient for exaggerated or diminished pharmacological effects.[62,138] Follow the directions in section 3.5.

Lercanidipine

Presentation
Film-coated tablets.

Administration - enteral tubes / swallowing difficulties
The tablets can be crushed and mixed with water for administration.[69] Follow the directions in section 3.5.

Levetiracetam

Presentation
Film-coated tablets.
Oral solution.

Administration - enteral tubes
1st choice – Use the oral solution. Follow the directions in section 3.6.
2nd choice – The tablets can be crushed and mixed with water for administration.[104,105] The active drug will dissolve but the excipients will not.[108] Follow the directions in section 3.5.

Administration - swallowing difficulties
1st choice – Use the oral solution. Follow the directions in section 3.6.
2nd choice – The tablets can be crushed and administered.[104,105] The active drug will dissolve but the excipients will not.[108] Follow the directions in section 3.5. Crushed levetiracetam tablets taste unpleasant. They can be diluted in orange juice to taste.[108]

Levofloxacin

Presentation
Tablets.
Infusion.

Administration - enteral tubes / swallowing difficulties
Give by infusion.

If infusion is not appropriate, consider changing to another quinolone such as ciprofloxacin. Levofloxacin tablets will not disperse.[70] Crushing them is not recommended, although this has been done in some centres.[132] Contact Pharmacy for advice.

Feed guidance
Levofloxacin will interact with sucralfate and antacids[35] and may interact with enteral feeds. If the tablets are administered enterally, the enteral feed should be withheld for one hour before and two hours after each dose.[155]

Levomepromazine (Methotrimeprazine)

Presentation
Tablets.
Injection.

Administration - enteral tubes / swallowing difficulties
1st choice – Consider giving by parenteral injection.
2nd choice – A suspension may be available in some centres.[95,169]
Follow the directions in section 3.6.
3rd choice – The tablets can be dispersed in water for administration if necessary.[102] They disperse immediately.[154] Follow the directions in section 3.5.
4th choice – The injection has also been used enterally.[104,164] Follow the directions in section 3.6.

Clinical guidance
Levomepromazine injection contains excipients which, when given enterally, degrade to products which theoretically may induce asthma attacks. No reports of attacks ever having been induced this way have been recorded by the manufacturers and the risk is considered to be small.[164]

Levothyroxine (Thyroxine)

Presentation
Tablets.

Administration - enteral tubes / swallowing difficulties
1st choice – A suspension can be made by Pharmacy at some centres. Dilute with the same volume of water before administering. Follow the directions in section 3.6.
2nd choice – The tablets can be crushed and mixed with water for administration.[152] Follow the directions in section 3.5.

Clinical guidance
Monitor thyroid function. There have been reports of treatment failure in patients receiving levothyroxine suspension, believed to be due to oxidation of the drug.[121,122] If thyroid function deteriorates, consider crushing tablets and mixing with water immediately prior to administration to reduce oxidation, or switching to liothyronine.

Feed guidance
Enteral feeds, especially soya based formulas, may increase faecal elimination of thyroxine.[87]

Linezolid

Presentation
Film-coated tablets.
Suspension.
Infusion.

Administration - enteral tubes
1st choice – Give by parenteral infusion if possible.
2nd choice – The tablets can be crushed and dispersed in water.[71]
Follow the directions in section 3.5.

The suspension may be too thick for administration through enteral feeding tubes.[132]

Administration - swallowing difficulties
1st choice – Give by parenteral infusion, or use the suspension.
2nd choice – The tablets can be crushed and dispersed in water.[71]
Follow the directions in section 3.5.

Clinical guidance
Monitor the patient for suitable effect.[71]

Lisinopril

Presentation
Tablets.
Sugar-free oral solution (special).

Administration - enteral tubes / swallowing difficulties
1st choice – The sugar-free oral solution (special) should be used if available.[129] Follow the directions in section 3.6.
2nd choice – A suspension can be made in Pharmacy in some centres. Dilute this with the same volume of distilled water, and flush post dose with 15-30ml of distilled water.
3rd choice – The tablets can be dispersed in water.[40,46] They disperse in one to five minutes.[154] Follow the directions in section 3.5.

Lisuride (Lysuride)

Presentation
Tablets.

Administration - enteral tubes / swallowing difficulties
The tablets can be crushed and mixed with water for administration.[41] Follow the directions in section 3.5.

Lithium

Presentation
Modified-release tablets.
Sugar-free oral liquid (some preparations contain sorbitol).

Administration - enteral tubes / swallowing difficulties
Use the equivalent dose of the liquid. Contact Pharmacy for advice on calculation of equivalent dose and monitoring of changeover. Follow the directions in section 3.6.

Clinical guidance
Lithium carbonate 200mg is approximately equivalent to lithium citrate 509mg, but different preparations of lithium vary widely in their bioavailability.[106] As most lithium tablets are modified-release, the total daily dose will need to be given in divided doses.

A change in lithium preparation usually requires the same precautions as initiation of treatment. Lithium concentration is affected by sodium, - an increase in serum sodium will result in increased lithium excretion, and therefore reduced lithium levels. Increases in lithium levels occur with sodium depletion / dehydration, or with a low salt diet. As lithium is highly toxic when serum levels rise a little above the normal treatment range, close monitoring is needed in these situations.

Feed guidance
Lithium absorption is decreased in the presence of enteral feeds. Feeds should be withheld for one hour before and two hours after each dose.[117]

Lofepramine

Presentation
Tablets.
Suspension (some preparations contain alcohol and / or sorbitol).

Administration - enteral tubes / swallowing difficulties
Use the suspension. Follow the directions in section 3.6.

The tablets are not suitable for crushing.[40]

Loperamide

Presentation
Capsule.
Liquid.

Administration - enteral tubes / swallowing difficulties
Use the liquid. Do not dilute. Follow the directions in section 3.6.

Clinical guidance
Do not open the capsules as they may cause enteral tube blockage and the bioavailability of the drug may be altered.

Loperamide liquid is suitable for administration through enteral tubes terminating in the jejunum. The liquid should be given undiluted to facilitate its dose dependant effect on motility. Flushing should still occur. The liquid has a very low osmolality and does not contain sorbitol and will therefore be tolerated.[17,158]

Loratadine

Presentation
Tablets.
Syrup.

Administration - enteral tubes / swallowing difficulties
Use the syrup.[94,104] Follow the directions in section 3.6.

Lorazepam

Presentation
Tablets.
Injection.

Administration - enteral tubes / swallowing difficulties
The tablets can be crushed and mixed with water for administration.[104,105] Without crushing they disperse in around five minutes.[154] Follow the directions in section 3.5. The tablets may also be effective if given sublingually,[105,152] but be aware that the patient must have a sufficiently moist mouth for this.

Lormetazepam

Presentation
Tablets.

Administration - enteral tubes / swallowing difficulties
The tablets can be dispersed in water for administration.[104] They disperse in one to five minutes.[154] Follow the directions in section 3.5.

Losartan

Presentation
Film-coated tablets.

Administration - enteral tubes / swallowing difficulties
The tablets can be crushed and mixed with water for administration.[63] Follow the directions in section 3.5.

Magnesium glycerophosphate

Presentation
Tablets.
Oral liquid.
Powder.

Administration - enteral tubes / swallowing difficulties
1st choice – Use the oral liquid.[140] Follow the directions in section 3.6.
2nd choice – The tablets can be crushed and mixed with water for administration.[132,152] Follow the directions in section 3.5.

Mebendazole

Presentation
Chewable tablets.
Suspension.

Administration - enteral tubes / swallowing difficulties
Use the suspension.[41,104] Follow the directions in section 3.6.

Mebeverine

Presentation
Tablets.
Liquid.
Modified-release capsules.

Administration - enteral tubes / swallowing difficulties
Use the liquid.[104] Follow the directions in section 3.6. Contact Pharmacy for advice about patients on the modified-release capsules.

150mg (15ml) liquid	equivalent to	135mg tablet[106]

Medroxyprogesterone

Presentation
Tablets.
Depot injection.
Injection.

Administration - enteral tubes / swallowing difficulties
The tablets can be crushed (preferably in water to reduce dust production) and mixed with water for administration.[66] Without crushing they disperse in around five minutes.[154] Use immediately. Follow the directions in section 3.5. Depo-Provera® has been used orally, but little data is available on this.[66]

Mefenamic acid

Presentation
Tablets, capsules.
Suspension.

Administration - enteral tubes / swallowing difficulties
Use the suspension.[104] Follow the directions in section 3.6.

Mefloquine

Presentation
Tablets.

Administration – enteral tubes
No information about the use of this medication via enteral feeding tubes has been located.

Administration – swallowing difficulties
The tablets can be crushed.[152]

Megestrol acetate

Presentation
Tablets.

Administration – enteral tubes
1st choice – A suspension can be made by Pharmacy in some centres. Follow the directions in section 3.6.
2nd choice – The tablets can be dispersed in water for administration.[68] The 40mg tablets disperse immediately.[154] The 160mg tablets disperse in one to five minutes.[154] Follow the directions in section 3.5. No information has been located on whether megestrol acetate is likely to block enteral feeding tubes.[68]

Administration – swallowing difficulties
1st choice – Use the Pharmacy-prepared suspension if available.
2nd choice – The tablets can be crushed and given in fruit juice or jam.[105] If the tablets are crushed this should preferably be done in water to reduce dust production.

Melatonin

Presentation
Capsules.
Modified-release capsules.

Administration - enteral tubes
The standard capsules can be opened and the contents mixed with water for administration.[105,152] Follow the directions in section 3.7.

Administration - swallowing difficulties
The standard capsules can be opened and the contents mixed with water, milk, yoghurt or fruit juice for administration.[105,152] Follow the directions in section 3.7.

Meloxicam

Presentation
Tablets.
Suppositories.

Administration - enteral tubes / swallowing difficulties
1st choice – Use the suppositories, or consider switching to an alternative non-steroidal anti-inflammatory drug.
2nd choice – The tablets can be crushed and dispersed in water for administration.[44,152] Follow the directions in section 3.5.

Menadiol

Presentation
Tablets.

Administration - enteral tubes / swallowing difficulties
The tablets can be crushed and mixed with water for administration.[104,105,152] Follow the directions in section 3.5. The crushed tablets have also been mixed with food for patients with swallowing difficulties.[132]

See also the entry under 'Phytomenadione'.

Meprobamate

Presentation
Tablets.

Administration - enteral tubes / swallowing difficulties
The tablets can be crushed and mixed with water for administration.[138] They are poorly soluble.[138] Follow the directions in section 3.5.

Meptazinol

Presentation
Tablets.
Injection.

Administration - enteral tubes / swallowing difficulties
1st choice – Give by parenteral injection if appropriate.
2nd choice - The tablets can be crushed and mixed with water for administration.[138] Follow the directions in section 3.5.

Mercaptamine

Presentation
Capsules.
Eye drops.

Administration – enteral tubes
No information about the use of this medication via enteral feeding tubes has been located.

Administration – swallowing difficulties
The capsules can be opened and the contents sprinkled on food or mixed in a strongly flavoured drink. The capsule contents have an unpleasant taste and smell. Do not mix with acidic drinks (i.e. orange juice etc.) as the drug may precipitate out.[152]

Mercaptopurine

Presentation
Tablets.

Administration - enteral tubes / swallowing difficulties
Caution – cytotoxic. Contact Pharmacy for advice before giving.
A suspension has been made by Pharmacy in some centres.[138]
Follow the directions in section 3.6.

Mesalazine

Presentation
Tablets.
Granules.
Foam enema.
Suppositories.

Administration – enteral tubes
The tablets are enteric-coated and designed for release in the small intestine. Do not crush. Consider rectal route if appropriate to the location of the condition, or an alternative drug.[94]

Pentasa® tablets will disperse in water, leaving small beads which must be swallowed / administered whole (so are therefore suitable only for larger bore tubes).[105,152]

Administration – swallowing difficulties
Consider rectal route if appropriate to the location of the condition.

The granules can be used for patients with swallowing difficulties. They should not be chewed, and therefore this method may not be appropriate for patients with limited understanding or impaired ability to follow instructions.

Alternatively Pentasa® tablets will disperse in water, leaving small beads which must be swallowed whole (so therefore may not be appropriate for patients with limited understanding or impaired ability to follow instructions).[105,152]

Metformin

Presentation
Tablets.
Modified-release tablets.
Sugar-free oral solution (special).

Administration - enteral tubes / swallowing difficulties
1st choice – Consider whether switching to insulin would be appropriate.
2nd choice – Use the oral solution if available. Follow the directions in section 3.6.
3rd choice – A suspension can be made up by Pharmacy at some centres. Follow the directions in section 3.6.

Do not crush the tablets.

Clinical guidance
Monitor blood glucose levels.

Methionine

Presentation
Tablets, capsules (special).

Administration – enteral tubes
No information about the use of this medication via enteral feeding tubes has been located.

Administration – swallowing difficulties
The capsules may be opened and the contents sprinkled onto food. The tablets should not be crushed.[152]

Methotrexate

Presentation
Tablets.
Injection.

Administration - enteral tubes / swallowing difficulties
<u>Caution – cytotoxic.</u> Contact Pharmacy for advice before giving.
A 'special' suspension may be available.[132] Follow the directions in
section 3.6.

The injection has also been given enterally in some centres, however
the manufacturers have no information on this, and cannot
recommend it.[40,167] Contact Pharmacy for advice.

Methylcellulose

Presentation
Tablets.

Administration - enteral tubes / swallowing difficulties
The tablets can be crushed and mixed with water for
administration.[138] Follow the directions in section 3.5.

Methyldopa

Presentation
Tablets.
Suspension.

Administration - enteral tubes / swallowing difficulties
1st choice – Use the suspension (if giving via enteral feeding tube, dilute with an equal volume of water).[132] Follow the directions in section 3.6.
2nd choice – The tablets can be crushed and mixed with water for administration.[133] Follow the directions in section 3.5.

Feed guidance
Methyldopa interacts with Ensure®, Ensure Plus®, and Osmolite® feeds, - feeds should be stopped for two hours before and one hour after administration of the medicine.[105]

Methylphenidate

Presentation
Tablets.
Modified-release tablets.

Administration - enteral tubes / swallowing difficulties
Use the standard tablets. Crush and mix with water for administration.[87] Follow the directions in section 3.5.

Do not crush the modified-release tablets.

Methylprednisolone

Presentation
Tablets.
Injections.
Intramuscular depot injection.

Administration - enteral tubes / swallowing difficulties
The tablets can be dispersed in water for administration.[105] They disperse within one minute.[154] Follow the directions in section 3.5.

Metoclopramide

Presentation
Tablets.
Modified-release tablets, modified-release capsules.
Oral solution (some preparations contain sorbitol).
Injection.

Administration - enteral tubes / swallowing difficulties
1st choice – Give by parenteral injection if possible.
2nd choice – Use the oral solution. Follow the directions in section 3.6.
3rd choice – The tablets have also been crushed and mixed with water for administration.[138] Follow the directions in section 3.5. Do not crush the modified-release tablets.
4th choice – The injection has been used enterally.[40,169] Follow the directions in section 3.6.

Metolazone

Presentation
Tablets.

Administration - enteral tubes / swallowing difficulties
The tablets can be crushed and mixed with water for administration.[104,105,152] Follow the directions in section 3.5.

Monitor the patient for postural hypotension due to increased bioavailability.[104] A dose reduction may be necessary.[135]

Metoprolol

Presentation
Tablets.
Modified-release tablets.
Suspension (special).
Injection.

Administration - enteral tubes / swallowing difficulties
1st choice - Consider giving by parenteral injection, or switching to an alternative beta-blocker available as a liquid.
2nd choice – Use the suspension if available.[138] Follow the directions in section 3.6.
3rd choice – A suspension can be made by Pharmacy at some centres. Dilute with the same volume of distilled water before administration. Follow the directions in section 3.6.
4th choice – The tablet can be crushed and mixed with water for administration. It disperses very slowly.[7,40] Follow the directions in section 3.5. Do not crush / disperse the modified-release tablets.

The injection has been given enterally at some centres, but there is very little information on this, so it is not recommended.[40,175] Contact Pharmacy for advice.

Metronidazole

Presentation
Tablets.
Suspension (metronidazole benzoate) (some preparations contain sorbitol).
Suppositories.
Intravenous infusion.

Administration – NG / PEG tubes / swallowing difficulties
1st choice – Give by intravenous infusion or rectally as suppositories when possible. Contact Pharmacy for advice on doses.
2nd choice – Use the suspension. Follow the directions in section 3.6.

Administration – NJ / PEJ / PEGJ tubes
1st choice – Give by intravenous infusion or rectally as suppositories when possible. Contact Pharmacy for advice on doses.
2nd choice – Crush the tablets in the case of patients with enteral tubes terminating in the jejunum, as the stomach acids are required to breakdown metronidazole benzoate to metronidazole. Without crushing the tablets disperse in around five minutes.[154] Follow the directions in section 3.5.

Clinical guidance
Metronidazole is well absorbed from the small intestines[66] and therefore it should be well absorbed when a suspension prepared from the tablets is administered to the jejunum.

Suppositories are unsuitable for the initiation of treatment of serious conditions owing to their slower absorption and lower plasma levels.[19] They are suitable to be used during ongoing treatment.

Feed guidance
The suspension should be administered one hour before food to allow metronidazole benzoate suspension to be broken down to metronidazole by the gastric enzymes in the stomach. Withhold enteral feeds for one hour before and one hour after each dose when the suspension is being used.[117]

Food affects the rate but not the extent of absorption of the tablets.[9,18]

Metyrapone

Presentation
Capsules.

Administration - enteral tubes / swallowing difficulties
The capsules can be opened, and the liquid contents squeezed out and dispersed in water for administration.[105,132] Beware of under-dosing due to not all the dose being obtained from the capsule. Follow the directions in section 3.7.

Mexiletine

Presentation
Capsules.
Injection.

Administration - enteral tubes / swallowing difficulties
1st choice – The capsules can be opened, and the contents dispersed in distilled water for administration.[105] Follow the directions in section 3.7.
2nd choice – The injection has also been administered enterally.[40,170] Follow the directions in section 3.6. It has a very unpleasant taste and a local anaesthetic action in the mouth.[170]

Feed guidance
When the injection is being given enterally to patients with swallowing difficulties, it should be given at least 30 minutes before food as it has a local anaesthetic effect.[40]

Mianserin

Presentation
Tablets.

Administration - enteral tubes / swallowing difficulties
The tablets can be dispersed in water for administration.[41,95] They disperse in one to five minutes.[154] Dispersed tablets may have a local anaesthetic effect on the mouth if given orally.[95] Follow the directions in section 3.5.

Midazolam

Presentation
Syrup.
Buccal liquid.
Injection.

Clinical guidance
Give by parenteral injection or infusion, or by the intranasal or buccal route.

Midodrine

Presentation
Tablets.

Administration - enteral tubes / swallowing difficulties
The tablets can be crushed and mixed with water for administration.[151] Follow the directions in section 3.5.

Minocycline

Presentation
Tablets, capsules.
Modified-release capsules.

Administration - enteral tubes / swallowing difficulties
1st choice – Switch to an alternative tetracycline antibiotic available as dispersible tablets (e.g. doxycycline) if possible.
2nd choice – The tablets can be crushed and mixed with water for administration.[138] Follow the directions in section 3.5.

The modified-release capsules have been opened and the contents given via enteral feeding tubes with plenty of water, but this is not recommended due to the risk of tube blockage. Do not crush the contents of the modified-release capsules.[138]

Minoxidil

Presentation
Tablets.

Administration - enteral tubes / swallowing difficulties
The tablets can be dispersed in water for administration.[40] They
disperse in one to five minutes.[154] Follow the directions in section
3.5. If giving via enteral feeding tube, flush well after each dose.

Mirtazepine

Presentation
Tablets.
Orodispersible tablets.
Oral solution.

Administration – enteral tubes
1st choice – Use the oral solution or the orodispersible tablets.
Follow the directions in sections 3.5 and 3.6. The orodispersible
tablets will disperse immediately in water.[154]
2nd choice – Crush the standard tablets well and mix with water for
administration.[72] The tablet may not fully dissolve, so take care to
flush the enteral tube well after administration. Follow the directions
in section 3.5.

Administration – swallowing difficulties
Use the oral solution or the orodispersible tablet, as the crushed
tablet has a bitter taste and an anaesthetic effect on the mouth.[72]
Follow the directions in section 3.6.

Misoprostol

Presentation
Tablets.

Administration - enteral tubes / swallowing difficulties
1st choice – Consider switching to an alternative medication which is available in a liquid or injection form, e.g. ranitidine, particularly if swallowing problems are likely to be long term, due to the hazards of handling dispersed tablets.
2nd choice – The tablets can be dispersed in water for administration.[104,105,152] They disperse immediately.[154] This should be done immediately before administration. Follow the directions in section 3.5.

Women who are or who may become pregnant should not handle crushed, broken, or dispersed tablets.[105]

Moclobemide

Presentation
Tablets.

Administration - enteral tubes / swallowing difficulties
The tablets can be crushed and dispersed in water for administration.[95] Follow the directions in section 3.5.

Montelukast

Presentation
Chewable tablets.
Film-coated tablets.
Granules.

Administration - enteral tubes / swallowing difficulties
Use the chewable tablets, and disperse in water for administration.[73]
Follow the directions in section 3.5.

Feed guidance
Withhold enteral feeds for two hours before and one hour after
administration of montelukast.[73]

Morphine

Presentation
Oral solution.
Film coated tablets.
Modified-release tablets, modified-release capsules, modified-
release sachets.
Suppositories.
Injection.

Administration – enteral tubes
Use parenteral morphine whenever possible. Consider
subcutaneous syringe drivers for chronic pain patients.

When an immediate release product is required, administer
morphine sulphate solution (e.g. Oramorph®). This is the preferred
enteral method of administering morphine. Follow the directions in
section 3.6.

When a controlled release product is required use MST Continus®
sachets, dilute with at least 30ml of water, and flush with 15-30ml of
distilled water. Give immediately as the resulting suspension
thickens. Alternatively, Zomorph® capsules can be opened and the
contents flushed down an enteral feeding tube with a diameter
greater than 16 French.[47,104]

(monograph continues on next page)

Administration – swallowing difficulties
Use MST Continus® sachets or the immediate release oral solution.

Zomorph® capsules can be opened, and their contents sprinkled onto food e.g. yoghurt or jam.[47,104]

MXL® capsules can also be opened and the contents sprinkled onto cold soft food for patients with swallowing difficulties.[146] The contents of the capsules should not be chewed or crushed, and therefore this method may not be appropriate for patients with limited understanding or impaired ability to follow instructions.

For patients with swallowing difficulties unable to receive morphine orally, the preferred alternative routes are rectally and subcutaneous. The bioavailabilty and duration of analgesia of morphine when given in the soluble, dispersible and rectal formulations are the same.[15]

Clinical guidance
The volume of water used for preparing the MST Continus® sachet does not affect the slow release properties of the beads in the sachets.

Do not administer MXL® capsules through enteral feeding tubes, as the granules in the capsules are highly lipophilic and will clump together when in contact with water or saline.[20]

Feed guidance
Morphine interacts with Jevity® feeds – withhold the feed for two hours before and one hour after each dose.[105]

Moxisylyte

Presentation
Film-coated tablets.

Administration - enteral tubes / swallowing difficulties
The tablets can be crushed and dispersed in water for administration.[138] Follow the directions in section 3.5.

Moxonidine

Presentation
Tablets.

Administration - enteral tubes / swallowing difficulties
The tablets can be crushed finely and dispersed in water for administration.[74] Without crushing they disperse in around five minutes.[154] Follow the directions in section 3.5.

The tablets are poorly soluble and film coated. They should be crushed well to minimise the risk of blocking enteral feeding tubes. The manufacturer recommends crushing one tablet and mixing it in 50ml of water, then allowing it to dissolve for 2 minutes before administering.[74]

Multivitamins

Presentation
Tablets.
Oral drops.

Clinical guidance
Consider whether vitamins are still required (vitamins are present in most enteral feeds). Use oral drops if necessary.

Mycophenolate mofetil

Presentation
Tablets, capsules.
Oral suspension.
Intravenous infusion.

Administration - enteral tubes / swallowing difficulties
1st choice – Use the intravenous infusion if possible at the same dosage as oral.[126]
2nd choice – The suspension can be given via enteral feeding tubes (minimum size 8 French).[127] Follow the directions in section 3.6.
3rd choice – The intravenous powder for injection has been used via enteral feeding tubes. The injection should be reconstituted as usual and administered via enteral feeding tube with a dextrose 5% flush before and after administration. Care should be taken when handling the powder (teratogenic risk).[126] Contamination should be removed promptly by washing with soap and water (eyes – plain water).[152]

Nabilone

Presentation
Capsules.

Administration - enteral tubes / swallowing difficulties
The capsules can be opened, and the contents dispersed in water for administration.[104] Give immediately. Follow the directions in section 3.7.

Nabumetone

Presentation
Tablets, film-coated tablets.
Dispersible tablets.
Suspension.

Administration - enteral tubes / swallowing difficulties
Use the suspension or the dispersible tablets. Follow the directions in section 3.6. The dispersible tablets may not be suitable for fine bore nasogastric tubes. Flush well after administration.[140]

Nadolol

Presentation
Tablets.

Administration - enteral tubes / swallowing difficulties
The tablets can be crushed and dispersed in water for administration.[138] Follow the directions in section 3.5.

Naftidrofuryl oxalate

Presentation
Capsules.

Administration – enteral tubes
The capsules can be opened and the contents dispersed in water for administration via enteral feeding tubes.[91] Follow the directions in section 3.7.

Administration – swallowing difficulties
The powder is irritant and anaesthetic to the mouth and throat.[105] There is a risk of oesophageal stricture if the capsules are opened for oral use in patients with swallowing difficulties. To avoid this, the patient should drink 4-5 glasses of water after each dose.[91] Review the need for this medication, - it is seldom practical to administer these volumes of water.[105]

Nalidixic acid

Presentation
Tablets.
Suspension (some preparations contain sorbitol).

Administration - enteral tubes / swallowing difficulties
Use the suspension.[138] Follow the directions in section 3.6.

Naproxen

Presentation
Tablets.
Enteric-coated tablets.
Suspension.

Administration - enteral tubes / swallowing difficulties
1st choice – Consider switching to an alternative non-steroidal anti-inflammatory drug available via a different route, e.g. rectal.
2nd choice – Use the suspension.[104] Follow the directions in section 3.6.

Nefopam

Presentation
Film-coated tablets.
Injection.

Administration - enteral tubes / swallowing difficulties
1st choice – Give by parenteral injection if appropriate.
2nd choice – A suspension can be made in Pharmacy in some centres.[138] Follow the directions in section 3.6.

The tablets should not be crushed.[150]

Neomycin

Presentation
Tablets.

Administration - enteral tubes / swallowing difficulties
The tablets can be crushed and mixed with water for administration.[105] Follow the directions in section 3.5.

Neostigmine

Presentation
Tablets.
Injection.

Administration - enteral tubes / swallowing difficulties
The tablets can be crushed and mixed with water for administration. They may not be suitable for narrow-bore tubes.[140] Follow the directions in section 3.5.

Nicardipine

Presentation
Capsules.
Suspension (special).
Modified-release capsules.

Administration - enteral tubes / swallowing difficulties
1st choice – Use the suspension if available.[138] Follow the directions in section 3.6.
2nd choice – The capsules can be opened, and the contents dispersed in orange juice for administration.[105] Follow the directions in section 3.7.

Do not open the modified-release capsules. Contact Pharmacy for advice.

Niclosamide

Presentation
Tablets (special).

Administration – enteral tubes
No information about the use of this medication via enteral feeding tubes has been located.

Administration – swallowing difficulties
The tablets can be crushed and dispersed in water or orange juice.[152]

Nicorandil

Presentation
Tablets.

Administration - enteral tubes / swallowing difficulties
The tablets can be crushed and mixed with water for administration.[62] Without crushing they disperse in around five minutes.[154] Some of the excipients in the tablets are insoluble, so take care to flush enteral tubes well after administration.[62] Follow the directions in section 3.5.

Nifedipine

Presentation
Capsules.
Modified-release tablets, modified-release capsules.

Administration - enteral tubes / swallowing difficulties
Use of immediate release nifedipine capsules for blood pressure control is no longer recommended due to the risk of rebound hypertension and tachycardia. Consider alternative methods of blood pressure control.

Take care – Risk of profound drop in blood pressure if nifedipine is given incorrectly. Contact Pharmacy for advice.

(monograph continues on next page)

When an immediate release product is required

1. When giving via enteral feeding tube, flush pre-dose with normal saline.
2. At the patient's bedside remove the liquid from the capsule using a green needle and withdraw the contents into a syringe. A 1ml syringe is ideal, as the contents are very viscous. A 5mg Adalat® capsule should contain 0.17ml and a 10mg capsule 0.34ml of solution.[147]
3. Administer immediately to the patient as nifedipine is light sensitive.[41] When giving via enteral feeding tube, flush the liquid down the enteral tube using normal saline not water, as nifedipine is poorly soluble in water.

Give immediately. Be aware that serious errors have occurred due to the use of needles and syringes to handle oral medication.

Alternatively the capsule can be given sublingually by the patient biting the capsule and the contents being administered sublingually. Consult with medical staff before doing this.

When a modified-release is required

Slow release capsules (e.g. Coracten®) can be opened and the contents flushed down enteral feeding tubes for administration.[89] The capsule contents should not be crushed. Be sure to flush the enteral tube well after dose administration. Adalat Retard® tablets have also been crushed and dispersed in water for enteral tube adminstration. This should not affect the modified-release properties, but small alterations in bioavailability may occur.[138]

Clinical guidance
Do not crush any tablets other than Adalat Retard® as they are modified-release. Nifedipine is very short acting. If a long acting preparation is substituted with a short acting preparation, side effects such as hypotension may occur, therefore monitor blood pressure more closely. Food may alter the rate but not the extent of absorption.

(monograph continues on next page)

Consider changing to a long acting calcium antagonist such as amlodipine.

Clinical guidance
Nifedipine absorption occurs entirely within the small intestine, but complete absoption following administration via enteral tubes terminating in the jejunum cannot be guaranteed, so blood pressure should be monitored.[158]

Nimodipine

Presentation
Tablets.
Infusion.

Administration - enteral tubes / swallowing difficulties
1st choice – Give by IV infusion if possible.
2nd choice – Crush the tablet down to a fine powder at the patients bedside, mix with water, and give immediately.[43] The tablets degrade rapidly once crushed and are light sensitive, so should be used immediately.[43] Check the patency of enteral tubes after administration as the film coating on nimodipine may block narrow bore tubes. Follow the directions in section 3.5.

Nitrazepam

Presentation
Tablets.
Suspension.

Administration - enteral tubes / swallowing difficulties
Use the suspension. Follow the directions in section 3.6.

Nitrofurantoin

Presentation
Tablets, capsules.
Modified-release capsules.
Suspension.

Administration - enteral tubes / swallowing difficulties
1st choice – Use the suspension.[105] Follow the directions in section 3.6.
2nd choice - Macrodantin® capsules have been opened.[104] Follow the directions in section 3.7. Do not open the modified-release capsules.
3rd choice – The tablets have been crushed and mixed with water for administration.[138] Follow the directions in section 3.5.

Nizatidine

Presentation
Capsules.
Injection.

Clinical guidance
Nizatidine capsules are not suitable to be used down enteral feeding tubes, as whilst the drug dissolves in water, the excipients do not and may coat and block the tube.[48] Consider changing to ranitidine if appropriate.

Norethisterone

Presentation
Tablets.

Administration - enteral tubes / swallowing difficulties
The tablets can be crushed (preferably in water to reduce production of dust) and mixed with water for administration.[94] Follow the directions in section 3.5.

Norfloxacin

Presentation
Tablets.

Administration - enteral tubes
The tablets can be crushed and mixed with water for administration.[105] Flush well as the drug is poorly soluble.[105] Light sensitive, so give immediately.[132] Follow the directions in section 3.5.

Administration - swallowing difficulties
The tablets can be crushed and mixed with water for administration.[105] The crushed tablets taste unpleasant.[105] Light sensitive, so give immediately.[132] Follow the directions in section 3.5.

Feed guidance
Withhold enteral feeds for one hour before and two hours after a dose, as absorption is decreased in the presence of feeds.[87]

Ofloxacin

Presentation
Tablets.
Infusion.

Administration - enteral tubes / swallowing difficulties
1st choice – Give by infusion if possible.
2nd choice – The tablets can be crushed and mixed with distilled water for administration.[105] Do not mix with tap water as chelation may occur with ions in the tap water (see under ciprofloxacin). Use distilled water for flushing enteral tubes post-dose.[105] Follow the directions in section 3.5.

Feed guidance
Withhold enteral feeds for one hour before a dose and two hours after each dose, as ofloxacin absorption is reduced in the presence of feeds.[105]

Olanzapine

Presentation
Film-coated tablets.
Orodispersible 'Velotab®' tablets.
Injection.

Administration – enteral tubes
Use Velotab® and disperse in water.[35,152] Follow the directions in section 3.5.

Administration – swallowing difficulties
The Velotab® can be placed on the tongue or dispersed in water, orange juice, apple juice, milk, or coffee.

Olanzapine may be irritant to the skin and eyes, so take precautions to avoid contact (e.g. wear gloves).[133]

Olsalazine

Presentation
Tablets, capsules.

Administration - enteral tubes / swallowing difficulties
The tablets can be crushed and mixed with water for administration.[105] Follow the directions in section 3.5. Some sources recommend the use of warm sterile water.[155] The capsules can be opened and their contents dispersed in water.[104,152] Follow the directions in section 3.7.

Omeprazole

Presentation
MUP tablets.
Capsules.
Injection.

Administration – enteral tubes
Give by parenteral injection if possible. Contact Pharmacy for advice. For large bore tubes, or when a switch is not appropriate, disperse the MUP tablet in water.[35]

Recommended method

1. Place the MUP tablet in the barrel of an oral syringe with 25ml of water and 5ml of air and shake to disperse it.[104,138] The granules left after dispersal should not be crushed.
2. Ensure the tip of the syringe has not been clogged.
3. Attach the syringe to the tube whilst keeping the tip upright to prevent clogging.
4. Administer the medication with repeated inversion of the syringe and shaking in order to disperse the contents.
5. When the fluid is gone from the syringe, a further 25ml of water and 5ml of air should be drawn up, and the process repeated.[138,148] Flush the tube very well after giving dose, as this medication is prone to blocking tubes.

Alternative method

1. For patients with nasogastric / gastrostomy tubes, administer 10ml of sodium bicarbonate 8.4% (not necessary for feeding tubes terminating in the jejunum).
2. Add the MUP tablet or the contents of an omeprazole capsule to 10ml of sodium bicarbonate 8.4% and wait for 10 minutes for a turbid solution to be obtained.[158] – Note, medicines should never be left unattended.
3. Administer via the enteral feeding tube, and flush immediately with plenty of water.

(monograph continues on next page)

Some sources recommend use of the alternative method for all patients with tubes terminating in the jejunum.[155]

Administration – swallowing difficulties
Disperse the MUP tablet in water, then mix this with orange / apple / pineapple juice, apple sauce, or yoghurt.[153]

Ondansetron

Presentation
Film-coated tablets.
Melt tablets.
Syrup (contains sorbitol)
Suppositories.
Injection.

Administration - enteral tubes / swallowing difficulties
1st choice – For acute use, consider giving by parenteral injection or using the suppositories.
2nd choice – Use the syrup.[40,104] Follow the directions in section 3.6.
3rd choice – The injection has been used enterally,[40,171] and this may be preferable for administration via enteral tubes terminating in the jejunum as the syrup contains sorbitol. The injection is acidic, so when giving via enteral feeding tube, flush well before and after each dose to prevent precipitation of the drug.[171] Follow the directions in section 3.6.

Orlistat

Presentation
Capsules.

Administration - enteral tubes / swallowing difficulties
Review whether this drug is still appropriate. Contact Dieticians for advice. If necessary, the capsules can be opened, and the contents dispersed in water for administration.[105]

Orphenadrine

Presentation
Sugar-coated tablets.
Solution (some preparations contain sorbitol).

Administration - enteral tubes / swallowing difficulties
Use the solution.[104] Follow the directions in section 3.6.

Oxcarbazepine

Presentation
Film-coated tablets.
Oral suspension.

Administration - enteral tubes / swallowing difficulties
Use the suspension.[132] Follow the directions in section 3.6.

Oxprenolol

Presentation
Coated tablets.
Modified-release tablets.

Administration - enteral tubes / swallowing difficulties
The tablets can be crushed and mixed with water for
administration.[105] The crushed tablets taste very bitter.[105] Follow
the directions in section 3.5.

Do not crush the modified-release tablets.

Oxprenolol is absorbed from both the small and the large intestine,
so it is predicted that administration directly into the jejunum should
produce a similar effect to oral administration.[158]

Oxybutynin

Presentation
Tablets.
Modified-release tablets.
Elixir.

Administration - enteral tubes / swallowing difficulties
1st choice – Use the elixir.[104] Follow the directions in section 3.6.
2nd choice – The tablets have been crushed and mixed with water for administration.[138] Follow the directions in section 3.5.

Do not crush the modified-release tablets.

Oxycodone

Presentation
Capsules.
Liquid, concentrate.
Injection.
Modified-release tablets.

Clinical guidance
1st choice – Contact Pharmacy for advice on appropriate management. Consider giving by parenteral injection if available, or switching to an alternative opiate available via a non-enteral route.
2nd choice – Use the liquid. Follow the directions in section 3.6.

Oxytetracycline

Presentation
Tablets.
Capsule.

Administration – enteral tubes
1st choice – Consider switching to doxycycline dispersible tablets.
2nd choice – The tablets have been crushed and mixed with water for administration down enteral feeding tubes.[105] Follow the directions in section 3.5.

Administration – swallowing difficulties
The tablets should not be crushed for administration to patients with swallowing difficulties due to the risk of oesophageal ulceration and oesophagitis.[105] Consider switching to doxycycline dispersible tablets.

Feed guidance
Oxytetracycline interacts with enteral feeds. Withhold feeds for one hour before and one hour after administration of each dose.[138]

Pancreatin

Presentation
Capsules.
Granules.

Administration – enteral tubes
Creon® capsules can be opened, and the contents dispersed in water for administration.[104] Do not crush the granules if they are being administered into the stomach (i.e. via a nasogastric or gastrostomy tube). If the granules are to be given via a tube terminating in the jejunum, the low pH of the stomach is bypassed, so the granules should be crushed, or dissolved in sodium bicarbonate (this must be prescribed), and mixed with the feed.[105,138]

The frequency of dosing may have to be altered according to the feed type and duration. One recommendation is that if giving with an enteral feed, half the dose should be given before the feed, and half after.[105] Contact Dieticians for advice.

Nutrizym® may block enteral feeding tubes, so its use is not recommended.[138]

Administration – swallowing difficulties
Creon® capsules can be opened and the contents mixed with soft food (the granules should not be chewed, therefore this may not be suitable for patients with limited understanding or impaired ability to follow instructions).[104]

Pantoprazole

Presentation
Enteric-coated tablets.
Injection.

Clinical guidance
Consider switching to lansoprazole 'Fastabs'. Contact Pharmacy for advice. A pantoprazole suspension may be available from Pharmacy at some centres.[155]

Paracetamol

Presentation
Tablets.
Soluble tablets.
Suspension (some preparations contain sorbitol).
Suppositories.

Administration - enteral tubes / swallowing difficulties
1st choice – Use the suppositories if possible.
2nd choice – Use the soluble tablets or the suspension.[104] Follow the directions in sections 3.5 and 3.6. The soluble tablets are preferable to the suspension which is hyperosmolar and may cause diarrhoea when administered via enteral tubes terminating in the jejunum. However the soluble tablets contain a lot of sodium which may be a problem in some patients.[104]

Paracetamol appears to have a similar absorption profile when administered directly into the jejunum as when given orally.[158]

Paroxetine

Presentation
Film-coated tablets.
Liquid.

Administration - enteral tubes
1st choice – Use the liquid, and dilute with an equal volume of water before administration as it is quite viscous.[104,155] Follow the directions in section 3.6.
2nd choice – The tablets can be crushed and mixed with water for administration. They must be crushed well and the tube flushed well as the tablets are film-coated.[105] Follow the directions in section 3.5.

Administration - swallowing difficulties
1st choice – Use the liquid.[104,155] Follow the directions in section 3.6.
2nd choice – The tablets can be crushed and mixed with water for administration. The crushed tablets are bitter and have a slight local anaesthetic effect.[105] Follow the directions in section 3.5.

Penicillamine

Presentation
Tablets.

Administration - enteral tubes / swallowing difficulties
The tablets can be crushed and mixed with water for administration.[133] Give immediately.[155] Follow the directions in section 3.5.

Feed guidance
Withhold enteral feeds for at least half an hour before and half an hour after each dose.[155]

Penicillin V

See entry under 'Phenyoxymethylpenicillin'.

Pentazocine

Presentation
Tablets, capsules.
Suppositories.
Injection.

Administration - enteral tubes / swallowing difficulties
1st choice – Use the suppositories or give by parenteral injection if possible.
2nd choice – The injection has been given enterally, mixed with orange juice immediately before administration.[40] Follow the directions in section 3.6.

Pentoxifylline (Oxpentifylline)

Presentation
Modified-release tablets.

Administration - enteral tubes / swallowing difficulties
This drug is formulated as a modified-release tablet to reduce the risk of it causing dyspepsia. If the patient has been on it for a long time and has not experienced this problem, then the tablet may be crushed and dispersed in water for administration.[138] Contact Pharmacy for advice. Follow the directions in section 3.5.

Do not crush the modified-release tablets.

Peppermint oil

Presentation
Enteric-coated capsules.

Clinical guidance
Peppermint water may be an alternative.[138] Contact Pharmacy for advice.

Peppermint oil capsules should not be broken open as the contents are irritant.[136]

Pergolide

Presentation
Tablets.

Administration – enteral tubes
The tablets will disperse in water.[75] They disperse in one to five minutes.[154] Be sure to flush well to ensure the whole dose is given.[138] Follow the directions in section 3.5.

Administration – swallowing difficulties
The tablets can be crushed and administered in jam or yoghurt.[105]

Pericyazine

Presentation
Tablets.
Syrup.

Administration - enteral tubes / swallowing difficulties
1st choice – Use the syrup.[41] Follow the directions in section 3.6.
2nd choice – The tablets can be crushed and mixed with water for administration.[132] Follow the directions in section 3.5.

Perindopril

Presentation
Tablets.

Administration - enteral tubes / swallowing difficulties
1st choice – A suspension can be made by Pharmacy in some centres (3 day expiry).[95] Follow the directions in section 3.6.
2nd choice – The tablets can be crushed and mixed with water for administration.[45] Follow the directions in section 3.5.

Perindopril may not be effective when administered through enteral tubes terminating in the jejunum due to decreased absorption.[155]

Feed guidance
Perindopril should be taken before food, so withhold enteral feeds for at least two hours before and two hours after administration.[76]

Perphenazine

Presentation
Sugar-coated tablets.
Sugar-free oral solution (special).

Clinical guidance
No information on the use of perphenazine via enteral feeding tubes has been obtained.

Pethidine

Presentation
Tablets.
Injection.

Administration - enteral tubes / swallowing difficulties
1st choice – Give by parenteral injection if possible, or switch to an alternative opiate available via a non-enteral route.
2nd choice – A liquid may be available in some centres.[140] Follow the directions in section 3.6.
3rd choice – The injection can be given enterally.[152] Follow the directions in section 3.6.

Phenelzine

Presentation
Film-coated tablets.

Administration - enteral tubes / swallowing difficulties
The tablets can be crushed and mixed with water for administration.[104,105] The drug is unstable in water, so give immediately.[41] Follow the directions in section 3.5.

Phenobarbital (Phenobarbitone)

Presentation
Tablets.
Elixir.

Administration - enteral tubes / swallowing difficulties
1st choice – Use the elixir. The elixir contains alcohol 38%.[106] If this is a problem, an alcohol-free 'special' preparation may be available from Pharmacy. Follow the directions in section 3.6.
2nd choice – The tablets may be crushed and mixed with water for administration.[152] Follow the directions in section 3.5.

Phenoxybenzamine

Presentation
Capsules.
Injection.

Administration- enteral tubes
The powder in the capsules is poorly soluble and may block enteral feeding tubes.[109] Therefore administration via enteral feeding tubes is not recommended.

Administration – swallowing difficulties
The powder has been removed from the capsules for oral administration in patients with swallowing difficulties.[152]

Phenoxymethylpenicillin

Presentation
Tablets.
Suspension.

Administration - enteral tubes / swallowing difficulties
1st choice – Use an intravenous antibiotic if possible.
2nd choice – Use the suspension. Follow the directions in section 3.6.

Feed guidance
Penicillin V interacts with enteral feeds leading to unpredictable absorption (30-80%). Consider using doses at the upper end of the normal range. Withhold the feed for one hour before and two hours after each dose.[90] This may not be practical due to the frequency of dosing. Contact Nutrition Team for advice.

Phenytoin

Presentation
Tablets, capsules, chewable tablets.
Suspension.
Injection.

Administration – NG / PEG tubes
1st choice – Give by parenteral injection if possible as enteral absorption is extremely unpredictable.[90]
2nd choice – Convert to phenytoin suspension, preferably as a single daily dose. Mix the phenytoin suspension with the same volume of distilled water to a minimise adsorption to tubing[21,22,23,24] and to improve tolerance to the suspension.[25,37] Flush the enteral tube with 30ml of distilled water before and after administration.

The tablets, capsules, and chewable tablets should not be opened / crushed.

Administration – NJ / PEJ / PEGJ tubes
Administering phenytoin directly into the jejunum is not recommended as the drug will be less effective.[37] The suspension is also hyperosmolar and may cause diarrhoea if given directly into the jejunum.[104] If jejunal administration cannot be avoided, particular care must be taken to observe patients closely, monitor plasma levels and adjust dose where appropiate.[11]

Administration – swallowing difficulties
1st choice – Give by parenteral injection or use the suspension.

The tablets, capsules and chewable tablets should not be opened / crushed.

Clinical guidance
The suspension should be shaken well before use to ensure dispersion. When changing from solid dosage forms to the liquid preparation, a dose conversion must occur, as there is a different salt of phenytoin in the liquid than in the tablet / capsule.[35]

(monograph continues on next page)

Phenytoin suspension 90mg (Phenytoin base)	equivalent to	Phenytoin tablets / capsules 100mg (Phenytoin sodium)[90]

If the volumes of phenytoin suspension to be administered are not practical the capsule may be opened and administered according to the general guidelines.[37]

Caution – Phenytoin suspension is available in two strengths (30mg/5ml and 90mg/5ml) and this has led to errors.
It is recommended to maintain patients on a single preparation (i.e. always on the same strength) and to use the 30mg/5ml for patients with enteral feeding tubes.

Phenytoin has a narrow therapeutic range and therefore the exact dose of phenytoin which the patient receives may be critical. Patient response and levels should be monitored carefully, especially after any changes in the feeding regime, as the dosage may require adjustment. Phenytoin is highly affected by albumin levels, and doses may require adjustment in patients with low albumin. Contact Pharmacy for advice.

Therapeutic plasma levels are 10-20mg/litre.[35]

Feed guidance
Phenytoin exhibits a particularly strong interaction with enteral feeds (especially Osmolite®, Isocal®, Ensure®, and Jevity®[105]). It is necessary to stop enteral feeds for two hours before and two hours after giving phenytoin suspension to enhance absorption, otherwise reduced serum levels can occur with loss of seizure control. [11,6,26,27]

Phosphate

Presentation
Effervescent tablets.
Joulies phosphate solution.
Injection, infusion.

Clinical guidance
Contact Dieticians for advice. Give a high-phosphate enteral /
parenteral feed if possible. Correct severe phosphate deficiency by
infusion with close monitoring of phosphate, potassium, and calcium.

Phytomenadione

Presentation
Sugar-coated tablets.
'Neonatal' injection.
'MM' injection.

Administration - enteral tubes / swallowing difficulties
Use the 'MM' injection, which is licensed for oral use (although not
for enteral tube administration). If giving via enteral feeding tube,
flush well after each dose.[40,104]

Pimozide

Presentation
Tablets.

Administration - enteral tubes / swallowing difficulties
The tablets can be crushed and mixed with water for
administration.[41] Follow the directions in section 3.5.

Pioglitazone

Presentation
Tablets.

Administration - enteral tubes / swallowing difficulties
1st choice – Consider whether switching to insulin would be appropriate.
2nd choice – The tablets can be crushed and mixed with water for administration.[138] Give immediately.[138] Follow the directions in section 3.5.

Piracetam

Presentation
Film-coated tablets.
Solution.

Administration - enteral tubes / swallowing difficulties
Use the solution.[41] Follow the directions in section 3.6.

Piroxicam

Presentation
Capsules.
Dispersible tablets.
'Melt' tablets.
Suppositories.
Injection.

Administration - enteral tubes / swallowing difficulties
1st choice – Give by parenteral injection or use the suppositories.
2nd choice – Use the dispersible tablets and dissolve in at least 50ml of water as they are very irritant.[41,133] Follow the directions in section 3.5.

Pizotifen

Presentation
Tablets.
Elixir.

Administration - enteral tubes / swallowing difficulties
1st choice – Use the elixir.[41,104] Follow the directions in section 3.6.
2nd choice – The tablets have been crushed and mixed with water for administration.[133] Follow the directions in section 3.5.

Potassium chloride

Presentation
Effervescent tablets.
Modified-release tablets.
Liquid (contains sorbitol).

Administration - enteral tubes
1st choice – Give potassium-containing intravenous fluids if possible (contact Pharmacy for advice).
2nd choice – Use Sando K® effervescent tablets, or Kay-Cee-L® liquid. Kay-Cee-L® liquid is highly concentrated and contains sorbitol so dilute with 60-90ml of water before administration.[9,155] Follow the directions in sections 3.5 and 3.6.

Do not crush Slow K®, which are modified-release tablets.

Administration - swallowing difficulties
Use Sando K® effervescent tablets, or Kay-Cee-L® liquid (contains sorbitol). Follow the directions in sections 3.5 and 3.6.

Do not crush Slow K®, which are modified-release tablets.

Pramipexole

Presentation
Tablets.

Administration - enteral tubes / swallowing difficulties
The tablets can be crushed and mixed with water for administration.[104,105] Follow the directions in section 3.5.

Pravastatin

Presentation
Tablets.

Administration - enteral tubes / swallowing difficulties
The tablets can be crushed and mixed with water for administration.[77] Use immediately.[77] Follow the directions in section 3.5.

Prazosin

Presentation
Tablets.

Administration - enteral tubes / swallowing difficulties
The tablets can be dispersed in water for administration.[104,105,152] The 500mcg tablet disperses immediately.[154] The 1mg tablet disperses within one minute.[154] The drug is very insoluble, so if giving via enteral feeding tube, flush well after each dose.[105] Follow the directions in section 3.5.

Prednisolone

Presentation
Tablets.
Enteric-coated tablets.
Soluble tablets.

Administration - enteral tubes / swallowing difficulties
Use the soluble tablets. Follow the directions in section 3.5.

Pregabalin

Presentation
Capsules.

Administration - enteral tubes / swallowing difficulties
Open the capsules and dissolve the contents in water for administration. The capsule contents may have an unpleasant taste.[125] Follow the directions in section 3.7.

Primaquine

Presentation
Tablets.

Administration - enteral tubes / swallowing difficulties
The tablets can be crushed and mixed with water for administration.[133] Follow the directions in section 3.5.

Primidone

Presentation
Tablets.
Liquid (unlicensed).

Administration - enteral tubes / swallowing difficulties
1st choice – Use the liquid.[41,104] Follow the directions in section 3.6.
2nd choice – The tablets can be crushed and dispersed in water for administration.[132] Follow the directions in section 3.5.

Probenecid

Presentation
Tablets.

Administration - enteral tubes / swallowing difficulties
The tablets can be crushed and mixed with water for administration.[133] Follow the directions in section 3.5.

Procainamide

Presentation
Tablets, capsules.
Injection.

Administration - enteral tubes / swallowing difficulties
1st choice – The tablets can be crushed and mixed with water for administration.[87] Follow the directions in section 3.5.
2nd choice – A suspension can be made at some centres.[173] Follow the directions in section 3.6.

The injection has been diluted 1:1 with syrup and given enterally in some centres, however there is little information available on this, so it is not recommended.[40] Contact Pharmacy for advice.

Procarbazine

Presentation
Capsules.

Administration - enteral tubes / swallowing difficulties
<u>Caution – cytotoxic.</u> Contact Pharmacy for advice before giving.

1st choice – A suspension may be made by Pharmacy in some centres.[138] Follow the directions in section 3.6.
2nd choice – The capsules are cytotoxic and should not be opened except on Pharmacy advice. If no other method is appropriate, on advice from Pharmacy the capsules can be opened and the contents administered in water or flushed down an enteral feeding tube with water. Give immediately as it is unstable. The powder is very irritant.[138] Follow the directions in section 3.7.

Prochlorperazine

Presentation
Tablets.
Buccal tablets.
Syrup, effervescent tablets.
Suppositories.
Injection.

Administration - enteral tubes / swallowing difficulties
1st choice – Give by parenteral injection, or use the buccal tablets or the suppositories if possible.
2nd choice – Use the syrup.[138] Follow the directions in section 3.6.

Procyclidine

Presentation
Tablets.
Syrup.
Injection.

Administration - enteral tubes / swallowing difficulties
1st choice – Give by parenteral injection if possible.
2nd choice – Use the syrup. Follow the directions in section 3.6.
3rd choice – A suspension may be prepared by Pharmacy in some centres.[152]

The injection has been used enterally at some centres, but there is very little information available on this, so it is not recommended.[40] Follow the directions in section 3.6.

Proguanil

Presentation
Tablets.

Administration - enteral tubes
The tablets can be crushed and mixed with water for administration.[104,105,132,152] Follow the directions in section 3.5.

Administration - swallowing difficulties
The tablets can be crushed and mixed with water, milk, or jam.[104,105,132,152] Follow the directions in section 3.5.

Promazine

Presentation
Coated tablets.
Solution.
Injection.

Administration - enteral tubes / swallowing difficulties
Use the solution.[104] Follow the directions in section 3.6.

Promethazine hydrochloride

Presentation
Film-coated tablets.
Elixir.
Injection.

Administration - enteral tubes / swallowing difficulties
Use the elixir.[94,104] Follow the directions in section 3.6.

Propafenone

Presentation
Film-coated tablets.

Administration - enteral tubes / swallowing difficulties
The tablets can be crushed and mixed in 5% glucose for
administration.[104,152] The crushed tablets may have a local
anaesthetic effect. If given orally, the mouth should be rinsed
afterwards to reduce this.[152]

Propantheline

Presentation
Sugar-coated tablets.

Administration - enteral tubes / swallowing difficulties
1st choice – A suspension can be made by Pharmacy in some
centres.[95,138] Follow the directions in section 3.6.
2nd choice – The tablets can be crushed and mixed with water for
administration.[105] The crushed tablets may have a bitter taste.[132]
Follow the directions in section 3.5.

Propranolol

Presentation
Tablets.
Modified-release capsules.
Oral solution.
Injection.

Administration - enteral tubes / swallowing difficulties
1st choice – Use the oral solution. Follow the directions in section 3.6.

The injection has been given enterally at some centres, mixed in raspberry syrup if given orally.[40] However there is little information available on this, so it is not recommended.[175] Contact Pharmacy for advice.

Do not crush / open modified-release preparations. Seek advice from Pharmacy.

Propylthiouracil

Presentation
Tablets.

Administration - enteral tubes / swallowing difficulties
The tablets can be crushed and mixed with water for administration.[104,105] Follow the directions in section 3.5.

Pseudoephedrine

Presentation
Tablets.
Elixir.

Administration - enteral tubes / swallowing difficulties
Use the elixir.[104] Follow the directions in section 3.6.

Feed guidance
Pseudoephedrine is incompatible with enteral feeds. Withhold feeds for one hour before a dose and two hours after.[41]

Pyrazinamide

Presentation
Tablets.

Administration - enteral tubes / swallowing difficulties
1st choice – A suspension can be made by Pharmacy in some centres. Dilute with the same volume of distilled water before administration. Follow the directions in section 3.6.
2nd choice – The tablets can be dispersed in water immediately before administration.[95] They disperse in one to five minutes.[154] Follow the directions in section 3.5.

Feed guidance
Withhold enteral feeds for thirty minutes before and one hour after each dose.[95]

Pyridostigmine

Presentation
Tablets.

Administration - enteral tubes / swallowing difficulties
1st choice – A liquid can be made by Pharmacy in some centres.[95]
Follow the directions in section 3.6.
2nd choice – The tablets can be crushed and mixed with water for
administration.[7,40,95] If giving via enteral feeding tube, flush well after
administering. Follow the directions in section 3.5.

Pyridoxine

Presentation
Tablets.

Administration - enteral tubes / swallowing difficulties
1st choice – A liquid can be made by Pharmacy in some centres.[95]
Follow the directions in section 3.6.
2nd choice – The tablets can be crushed and mixed with water for
administration.[104,105] The 50mg tablets disperse in one to five
minutes.[154] Follow the directions in section 3.5.

Pyrimethamine

Presentation
Tablets.

Administration - enteral tubes / swallowing difficulties
The tablets can be crushed and mixed with water or juice for
administration.[40,152] Follow the directions in section 3.5.

Quetiapine

Presentation
Tablets.

Administration – enteral tubes
Quetiapine tablets are not soluble.[46] Contact Pharmacy for advice.
The tablets can be crushed and mixed with water for administration.
Flush well after administration.[105,134] Follow the directions in section
3.5.

Administration – swallowing difficulties
The crushed tablets have been added to soft food (e.g.
yoghurt).[105,134] They taste bitter.[134]

Quinidine

Presentation
Tablets.
Modified-release tablets.

Administration - enteral tubes / swallowing difficulties
The standard tablets can be crushed and mixed with water for
administration.[87] Follow the directions in section 3.5.

Do not crush the modified-release tablets. Contact Pharmacy for
advice on altering the dosage.

Quinine sulphate

Presentation
Tablets.

Administration - enteral tubes
Crush the tablets well, and disperse in a large volume (e.g. 200ml) of water. Flush well to minimise blockage and irritancy, as the coating is likely to block narrow-bore enteral feeding tubes.[78] Only use if absolutely necessary and swallowing problems are likely to be long term. Follow the directions in section 3.5.

Administration - swallowing difficulties
Crush the tablets well, and disperse in a large volume (e.g. 200ml) of water.[78] The crushed tablets have a bitter taste which may be masked by mixing with syrup.[105] Only use if absolutely necessary and swallowing problems are likely to be long term. Follow the directions in section 3.5.

Rabeprazole

Presentation
Enteric-coated tablets.

Clinical guidance
Crushing is not recommended as stomach acid can destroy the active drug.[105] Consider switching to lansoprazole 'Fastabs'. Contact Pharmacy for advice.

Raloxifene

Presentation
Tablets

Clinical guidance
The tablets should be discontinued if the patient is immobile, and are therefore probably unsuitable for use in most enteral tube fed patients.[75] Contact Pharmacy for advice on alternatives.

Ramipril

Presentation
Tablets, capsules.

Administration – enteral tubes
The capsules can be opened, and the contents dispersed in water for enteral tube administration.[62] Follow the directions in section 3.7.

The tablets can be crushed and dispersed in water for administration.[107] Follow the directions in section 3.5.

Administration – swallowing difficulties
The capsule contents can be placed directly into the mouth, or onto bread if the patient has swallowing difficulties.[62]

The capsule contents taste unpleasant.[62]

Ranitidine

Presentation
Tablets.
Effervescent tablets.
Syrup (some preparations contain alcohol and / or sorbitol).
Injection.

Administration - enteral tubes / swallowing difficulties
1st choice – Use the effervescent tablets, dissolved in at least 75ml water. Follow the directions in section 3.5.
2nd choice – Use the syrup. Follow the directions in section 3.6.
3rd choice – The injection can be administered through enteral feeding tubes to achieve therapeutic levels.[31,158] Follow the directions in section 3.6.

Clinical guidance
Absorption is most pronounced in the duodenum, followed by the jejunum and ileum. A negligible amount of drug is absorbed from the stomach.[28,29] Thus, ranitidine will be suitable for administration through enteral tubes terminating in the jejunum.[158] Absorption is not affected by the presence of food.[30]

The syrup is an alternative to the effervescent tablets. It is however more viscous and may block the enteral feeding tube. It also contains alcohol and sorbitol.

Reboxetine

Presentation
Tablets.

Administration - enteral tubes / swallowing difficulties
The tablets can be crushed and mixed with water for administration.[104,105] Follow the directions in section 3.5.

Repaglinide

Presentation
Tablets.

Administration - enteral tubes / swallowing difficulties
1st choice – Consider whether switching to insulin would be appropriate.
2nd choice – The tablets can be crushed and mixed with water for administration.[105] Follow the directions in section 3.5.

Monitor the patient's blood glucose. Repaglinide is absorbed faster in the duodenum than the stomach.[105]

Rifampicin

Presentation
Capsules.
Syrup.

Administration - enteral tubes / swallowing difficulties
Use the syrup (and when giving via enteral feeding tube, dilute with an equal volume of water before administration).[132] Follow the directions in section 3.6.

Feed guidance
Withhold enteral feeds for one hour before and one hour after administration, as rifampicin needs to be given on an empty stomach.[35,117]

Combination Products

Use the separate components if possible. If the components are not available, Rifater® and Rimactazid® brands have been crushed and mixed with water for administration.[105,133]

Riluzole

Presentation
Film-coated tablets.

Administration – enteral tubes
The tablets can be crushed and dispersed in water for enteral tube administration.[79] Give immediately. Follow the directions in section 3.5.

Administration – swallowing difficulties
The tablets can be crushed and mixed with soft food e.g. yoghurt or puree, to aid swallowing.[79] Tablets crushed onto food should be eaten within fifteen minutes as there is no stability data available for this method of administration.[79] Use crushed tablets with care as they may have a local anaesthetic effect in the mouth.[79]

Absorption may be affected by fatty food.[150]

Risedronate

Presentation
Tablets

Clinical guidance
Not suitable for crushing due to gastrointestinal side effects.[80]
Contact Pharmacy to discuss alternatives.

Risperidone

Presentation
Film-coated tablets.
Orodispersible tablets.
Liquid.
Depot injection.

Administration - enteral tubes / swallowing difficulties
Use the liquid or the orodispersible tablet.[104,132] Follow the directions in sections 3.5 and 3.6.

Ritonavir

Presentation
Capsules.
Solution.

Administration - enteral tubes
1st choice – Use the solution.[40] Follow the directions in section 3.6.
2nd choice – The capsules can be opened and the contents mixed with water for administration.[40,132] Follow the directions in section 3.7.

Administration - swallowing difficulties
1st choice – Use the solution.[40] Follow the directions in section 3.6.
2nd choice – The capsules can be opened and the contents mixed with water for administration. This has an extremely bad taste, which may be masked by chocolate milk.[40,132] Follow the directions in section 3.7.

Rivastigmine

Presentation
Capsules.
Solution.

Administration - enteral tubes / swallowing difficulties
1st choice – Use the solution if available. Follow the directions in section 3.6.
2nd choice – The capsules can be opened, and the contents dispersed in water for administration.[104,138] Follow the directions in section 3.7.

Ropinirole

Presentation
Film-coated tablets.

Administration – enteral tubes
The tablets can be crushed and mixed with water for administration via enteral feeding tubes.[81] Follow the directions in section 3.5. There is no information available to indicate whether ropinirole tablets are likely to block enteral feeding tubes.[81]

Administration – swallowing difficulties
The tablets can be crushed and mixed with soft food for patients with swallowing difficulties.[105]

Rosiglitazone

Presentation
Tablets.

Administration - enteral tubes / swallowing difficulties
1st choice – Consider whether switching to insulin would be appropriate.
2nd choice – The tablets can be crushed and dispersed in water for administration.[67] Follow the directions in section 3.5. No information has been located on whether rosiglitazone is likely to block enteral feeding tubes.[67]

Rosuvastatin

Presentation
Film-coated tablets.

Administration - enteral tubes / swallowing difficulties
The tablets can be crushed and mixed with water for administration.[150] Follow the directions in section 3.5.

Salbutamol

Presentation
Various preparations for inhalation.
Oral solution.
Tablets.
Modified-release tablets.
Injection.

Administration - enteral tubes / swallowing difficulties
1st choice – Use the oral solution. Follow the directions in section 3.6.
2nd choice – The standard tablets have been crushed and mixed with water for administration.[138,152] Follow the directions in section 3.5.

Do not crush the modified-release tablets.

Clinical guidance
If changing from sustained release tablets to the oral solution, a change in dose and frequency will be required. The oral solution should be given in three to four divided doses. Do not crush the sustained release tablets. Consider managing the patient with inhaled therapy (e.g. nebules).

Saquinavir

Presentation
Gel-filled capsules.
Capsules.

Administration - enteral tubes / swallowing difficulties
The capsules can be opened, and the gel contents dispersed in water for administration. The drug has a very bitter taste.[40] Follow the directions in section 3.7.

Secobarbital

Presentation
Capsules.
Powder.

Administration – enteral tubes
No information about the use of this medication via enteral feeding
tubes has been located.

Administration – swallowing difficulties
The powder can be administered in neat blackcurrant juice to
disguise the very bitter taste.[152]

Selegiline

Presentation
Tablets.
Liquid.
Lyophilisates.

Administration - enteral tubes / swallowing difficulties
1st choice – Use the liquid,[41,104,105] or the lyophilisate if the patient has
a moist mouth.[132] Follow the directions in section 3.6.
2nd choice – The tablets can be dispersed in water for
administration.[7] They disperse within one minute.[154] Follow the
directions in section 3.5.

Senna

Presentation
Tablets.
Syrup.

Administration - enteral tubes / swallowing difficulties
Use the syrup and flush post-dose with 15-30ml of distilled water.
Follow the directions in section 3.6.

Sertraline

Presentation
Tablets.

Administration – enteral tubes
The tablets can be dispersed in water for administration. They disperse in one to five minutes.[154] Follow the directions in section 3.5.

Administration – swallowing difficulties
The tablets can be crushed and mixed with food for patients with swallowing difficulties.[37,152] Crushed tablets have a bitter taste, and an anaesthetic effect on the tongue, so use with caution and take care with hot foods after administration.[37]

Clinical guidance
Consider changing to an alternative drug available as a syrup (e.g. fluoxetine, paroxetine) if swallowing problem is likely to be long term. Contact Pharmacy for advice.

Sildenafil

Presentation
Film-coated tablets.

Administration - enteral tubes / swallowing difficulties
The tablets can be crushed and dispersed in water for administration.[155] Follow the directions in section 3.5.

Simeticone

Presentation
Various combination preparations.

Administration - enteral tubes / swallowing difficulties
The drops can be administered via enteral feeding tubes.[87]

Simvastatin

Presentation
Tablets.

Administration - enteral tubes / swallowing difficulties
The tablets can be crushed and mixed with water for administration.[63] Use immediately (light sensitive).[63.95] Follow the directions in section 3.5.

Sodium bicarbonate

Presentation
Tablets, capsules.
Intravenous injection, infusion.

Administration - enteral tubes / swallowing difficulties
1st choice – The capsules can be opened and the contents mixed with water for administration.[144] Follow the directions in section 3.7.
2nd choice – The injection can be given enterally.[152] Follow the directions in section 3.6.

Sodium chloride

Presentation
Capsules (special).
Modified-release tablets.
Oral solution (special).
Injection.

Administration - enteral tubes / swallowing difficulties
1st choice – Use the oral solution if available. Follow the directions in section 3.6.
2nd choice – The injection can be given enterally.[152] Follow the directions in section 3.6.

Sodium clodronate

Presentation
Capsules.
Film-coated tablets.
Infusion.

Administration - enteral tubes / swallowing difficulties
The capsules can be opened and the contents dispersed in water for administration.[95,104] Follow the directions in section 3.7. Only mix with water; do not mix with calcium containing preparations e.g. milk, or other medicines.[95]

Feed guidance
Withhold enteral feeds for two hours before and two hours after each dose.[104]

Sodium cromoglicate (Sodium cromoglycate)

Presentation
Capsules.
Inhaler, nebules.
Eye drops.
Nasal spray.

Administration - enteral tubes / swallowing difficulties
The capsule contents can be removed, dissolved in warm water, and then diluted with cold water before administration.[138,152]

Sodium fusidate

Presentation
Enteric-coated tablets.
Suspension (contains sorbitol).
Intravenous infusion.

Administration - enteral tubes / swallowing difficulties
1st choice – Use the intravenous infusion if possible.
2nd choice – Use the suspension. Follow the directions in section 3.6.

| 750mg suspension | equivalent to | 500mg tablet[90] |

Sodium phenylbutyrate

Presentation
Tablets.
Suspension, granules.
Powder.
Injection.

Administration – enteral tubes
No information about the use of this medication via enteral feeding tubes has been located.

Administration – swallowing difficulties
The injection can be given orally.[152]

Sodium picosulfate (Sodium picosulphate)

Presentation
Capsules.
Elixir, sachets.

Administration - enteral tubes / swallowing difficulties
Use the elixir.[104] Follow the directions in section 3.6.

Sodium valproate

Presentation
Sugar-free oral liquid.
Tablets.
Crushable tablets.
Modified-release tablets.
Injection.

Administration - enteral tubes / swallowing difficulties
1st choice – Give by parenteral injection if possible. Contact Pharmacy for advice.
2nd choice – Use the liquid (contains sorbitol). Contact Pharmacy for advice on the appropriate dosage. The liquid should not be diluted.[155] Follow the directions in section 3.6.

Contact Pharmacy for advice on dose conversion, and if patient has previously been receiving Epilim Chrono®.

Sotalol

Presentation
Tablets.
Injection.

Administration - enteral tubes / swallowing difficulties
1st choice – Consider switching to an alternative beta-blocker available as a liquid.
2nd choice – A suspension can be prepared by Pharmacy at some centres. Follow the directions in section 3.6.
3rd choice – The tablet can be crushed and mixed with water for administration.[68,152] Follow the directions in section 3.5.

Spironolactone

Presentation
Tablets.
Sugar-free oral suspension (special).

Administration - enteral tubes / swallowing difficulties
1st choice – Use the suspension.[104] Follow the directions in section 3.6.
2nd choice – The tablets can be crushed and mixed with water for administration.[138,152] Follow the directions in section 3.5.

Stanozolol

Presentation
Tablets.

Administration - enteral tubes / swallowing difficulties
The tablet can be crushed and mixed with water for administration.[133] Follow the directions in section 3.5.

Stavudine

Presentation
Capsules.
Oral solution.

Administration - enteral tubes / swallowing difficulties
Use the oral solution.[138] Follow the directions in section 3.6.

Sucralfate

Presentation
Tablets.
Suspension.

Administration – NG / PEG tubes / swallowing difficulties
Review choice of drug as large breaks in feeding are required for administration of sucralfate. If essential, use the suspension and dilute well.[41]

Administration – NJ / PEJ / PEGJ tubes
Do not give. Sucralfrate is ineffective by this route. For treatment of duodenal and gastric ulcers and chronic gastritis, it is recommended to use ranitidine effervescent tablets.

Clinical guidance
Sucralfate may affect the absorption of other drugs, so administration of other medications should be separated from the sucralfate dosage by at least two hours.[155]

Feed guidance
Sucralfrate is the most frequent cause of obstruction of enteral feeding tubes[20] therefore it must be administered with particular care. The aluminium in sucralfate interacts with proteins in enteral feeds to form an insoluble precipitate (bezoar formation).[32]

An enteral feeding break of one hour before and one hour after administration of sucralfate is recommended.

Sulfasalazine (Sulphasalazine)

Presentation
Tablets.
Enteric-coated tablets.
Suspension.
Suppositories.
Retention enema.

Administration - enteral tubes / swallowing difficulties
1st choice – Consider using the suppositories or the enema for lower-bowel disease.
2nd choice – Use the suspension.[104,105] Follow the directions in section 3.6.

Sulindac

Presentation
Tablets.

Administration - enteral tubes / swallowing difficulties
The tablet can be crushed and mixed with water for administration.[133] Follow the directions in section 3.5.

Sulpiride

Presentation
Tablets.
Solution.

Administration - enteral tubes / swallowing difficulties
1st choice – Use the solution.[104,105] Follow the directions in section 3.6 25.
2nd choice – The tablets can be dispersed in water for administration.[41] They disperse in one to five minutes.[154] Follow the directions in section 3.5.

Tacrolimus

Presentation
Capsules.
Concentrate for infusion.

Administration - enteral tubes / swallowing difficulties
1st choice – Consider switching to the infusion.
2nd choice – The capsules can be opened and the contents dispersed in water for administration.[111] The carer should wear a mask and gloves when doing this to reduce exposure to the powder. Follow the directions in section 3.7.

Tamoxifen

Presentation
Tablets.
Solution (some preparations contain alcohol and / or sorbitol).

Administration – enteral tubes
1st choice – Use the solution.[104,105] Follow the directions in section 3.6.
2nd choice – The tablets can be crushed and mixed with water for administration.[94,105] Handle with care (see clinical guidance below). Follow the directions in section 3.5.

Administration – swallowing difficulties
The crushed tablets can be mixed with jam or yoghurt for patients with swallowing difficulties.[105] Handle with care (see clinical guidance below).

Clinical guidance
Handle the crushed tablets with care. Avoid the dust being inhaled, coming into contact with the skin, etc.[105] The carer should wear gloves, mask, and eye protection when crushing tablets.

Tamsulosin

Presentation
Capsules.
Film-coated modified-release tablets.

Clinical guidance
The tablet is modified-release and should not be crushed. The capsule is modified-release and is not suitable for opening for tube administration,[82] although this has been done. Contact Pharmacy for advice.

The capsules contain granules which should not be crushed. If no alternative is suitable, they may be mixed with cold water and swallowed whole (only suitable for patients able to follow the instruction not to chew) or given down an enteral feeding tube with good post-dose flushing.[105]

Telmisartan

Presentation
Tablets.

Administration - enteral tubes / swallowing difficulties
The tablets are only sparingly soluble but there are anecdotal reports of them being crushed and mixed with water for administration. If giving via enteral feeding tube, flush well after administration.[110] Follow the directions in section 3.5.

Temazepam

Presentation
Tablets.
Elixir (some preparations contain alcohol and / or sorbitol).

Administration - enteral tubes / swallowing difficulties
Use the elixir. Do not dilute. Follow the directions in section 3.6.

The tablets should not be used. They are quite insoluble and their use may lead to the blockage of enteral feeding tubes.

Clinical guidance
Temazepam may be less effective when administered through enteral tubes terminating in the jejunum.

Tenofovir

Presentation
Film-coated tablets.

Administration - enteral tubes / swallowing difficulties
The tablets can be dispersed in half a glass of water or orange juice for administration.[132] Follow the directions in section 3.5.

Terazosin

Presentation
Tablets.

Administration - enteral tubes / swallowing difficulties
The tablets can be dispersed in water for administration. They disperse in one to five minutes.[154] The excipients may not dissolve so it may be necessary to filter them out to prevent blockage of enteral feeding tubes.[56] Follow the directions in section 3.5.

Terbinafine

Presentation
Tablets.

Administration - enteral tubes / swallowing difficulties
1st choice – A suspension can be prepared by Pharmacy at some centres.[155] Follow the directions in section 3.6.
2nd choice – The tablets can be crushed and mixed with water for administration.[41] Follow the directions in section 3.5.

Tetrabenazine

Presentation
Tablets.

Administration - enteral tubes / swallowing difficulties
The tablets can be crushed and mixed with water for administration.[104] Flush well after administration.[132] Follow the directions in section 3.5.

Tetrahydrobiopterin

Presentation
Tablets.

Administration – enteral tubes
No information about the use of this medication via enteral feeding tubes has been located.

Administration – swallowing difficulties
The tablets may be dispersed in water or orange juice immediately before administration.[152]

Thalidomide

Presentation
Capsules.

Clinical Guidance
Thalidomide is not suitable for administration via enteral feeding tubes.[138]

Theophylline

Presentation
Liquid, sugar-free oral solution (special) (may be hard to obtain).
Tablets.
Various modified-release preparations.

Administration - enteral tubes / swallowing difficulties

When an immediate release preparation is required

1st choice – Dilute the liquid with distilled water.
2nd choice – Crush Nuelin® tablets and disperse in water for administration.[152] Follow the directions in section 3.5.

When a slow release preparation is required

It is recommended to switch to an immediate release preparation, but if a slow release preparation is needed, the following method can be used.

Open a Slo-phyllin® capsule and pour the contents, (enteric-coated granules) through the feeding tube, flushing before and after with 15-30ml of distilled water. The granules have also been administered on soft food for patients with swallowing difficulties.[132] The granules should not be chewed or crushed, and therefore this method may not be appropriate for patients with limited understanding or impaired ability to follow instructions.

(monograph continues on next page)

Do not crush the modified-release tablets.

Clinical guidance
There is a difference in bioavailability between the liquid and the modified-release tablets. The liquid should be given more frequently. Contact Pharmacy for advice on equivalent doses.

Additional notes
Aminophylline is a salt of theophylline. Patients on aminophylline tablets can be converted to theophylline hydrate liquid. This will require a dosage change. Contact Pharmacy for advice.

250mg oral aminophylline equivalent to 200mg oral theophylline[176]

Feed guidance
Administer theophylline on an empty stomach as it will interact with enteral feeds,[41] particularly Osmolite®, Ensure® and Ensure Plus®.[105] The patient should be monitored for loss of efficacy. Withhold enteral feeds for one hour before and two hours after each dose.[87,117]

Thiamine

Presentation
Tablets.

Administration - enteral tubes / swallowing difficulties
1st choice – A suspension can be prepared by Pharmacy at some centres. Follow the directions in section 3.6.
2nd choice – The tablets can be crushed and dispersed in water for administration.[94] Follow the directions in section 3.5.

Thioridazine

Presentation
Film-coated tablets.
Syrup (special), sugar-free oral solution (special).

Clinical guidance
The syrup has been administered in some centres, but there is little information available on this.[133] Follow the directions in section 3.6. No information on crushing the tablets has been located, so they should not be crushed.

Tiabendazole

Presentation
Tablets (special).
Syrup, suspension (special).

Administration – enteral tubes
No information about the use of this medication via enteral feeding tubes has been located.

Administration – swallowing difficulties
The tablets may be crushed for administration.[152]

Tiagabine

Presentation
Film-coated tablets.

Administration - enteral tubes / swallowing difficulties
The tablets can be crushed and mixed with water for administration.[104] Follow the directions in section 3.5.

Tinidazole

Presentation
Film-coated tablets.

Administration - enteral tubes / swallowing difficulties
The tablets can be crushed and dispersed in water for administration.[132] They have a very bitter taste which can be disguised with strongly flavoured juice when being administered to patients with swallowing difficulties.[132] Follow the directions in section 3.5.

Tioguanine (Thioguanine)

Presentation
Tablets.

Administration - enteral tubes / swallowing difficulties
Caution – cytotoxic. Contact Pharmacy for advice before giving. A suspension can be made by Pharmacy in some centres.[138] Follow the directions in section 3.6.

Tizanidine

Presentation
Tablets.

Administration - enteral tubes / swallowing difficulties
1st choice – A suspension is available from Pharmacy at some centres.[155] Follow the directions in section 3.6.
2nd choice – The tablets can be crushed and mixed with water for administration.[104] Follow the directions in section 3.5.

Tolbutamide

Presentation
Tablets.

Administration - enteral tubes / swallowing difficulties
1st choice – Consider whether switching to insulin would be appropriate.
2nd choice – The tablets can be crushed and mixed with water for administration.[104,105] Follow the directions in section 3.5.

Monitor the patient's blood glucose.

Tolterodine

Presentation
Tablets.
Modified-release capsules.

Administration - enteral tubes / swallowing difficulties
The tablets can be dispersed in water for administration.[83] They disperse within one minute.[154] Use immediately. Follow the directions in section 3.5. No information has been located to indicate whether tolterodine is likely to block enteral feeding tubes.[83]

The modified-release capsules contain time-release beads which can be removed from the capsule and administered whole, to patients with the ability to follow the instruction not to chew,[105] but the preferred form of tolterodine for administration is the standard tablets. Contact Pharmacy for advice.

Topiramate

Presentation
Tablets.
Sprinkle capsules.

Administration - enteral tubes
1st choice – The sprinkle capsules can be opened and the contents sprinkled on food or mixed with water and flushed down an enteral feeding tube (some sources do not recommend use via feeding tube[155]). Flush well to prevent blockage.[101] Follow the directions in section 3.7.
2nd choice – The tablets can be crushed and dispersed in water for administration.[95,152] Follow the directions in section 3.5.

Administration - swallowing difficulties
1st choice – The sprinkle capsules can be opened and the contents sprinkled on food or mixed with water for administration.[101] Follow the directions in section 3.7.
2nd choice – The tablets can be crushed and dispersed in water for administration.[95,152] Has a bitter taste if administered orally.[95,152] Follow the directions in section 3.5.

Torasemide

Presentation
Tablets.

Administration - enteral tubes / swallowing difficulties
The tablets can be crushed and dispersed in water for administration. A slurry may be formed, so if giving via enteral feeding tube, flush well after administration.[138] Follow the directions in section 3.5.

Tramadol

Presentation
Capsules.
Soluble tablets, orodispersible tablets, sachets, sugar-free oral solution (special).
Modified-release tablets, modified-release capsules.
Injection.

Administration - enteral tubes / swallowing difficulties
1st choice – For acute situations, consider giving by parenteral injection.
2nd choice – Use the soluble tablets, orodispersible tablets, or the oral solution. Follow the directions in sections 3.5 and 3.6.

Trandolapril

Presentation
Capsules.

Administration – enteral tubes
The capsules can be opened, and the contents dispersed in water for administration.[105] Follow the directions in section 3.7.

Administration – swallowing difficulties
The capsule contents have a bitter taste which can be masked by fruit squash for patients with swallowing difficulties.[155]

Tranexamic acid

Presentation
Tablets.
Injection.

Administration - enteral tubes / swallowing difficulties
1st choice – The tablets can be crushed and mixed with water for administration. Follow the directions in section 3.5.
2nd choice – The injection can also be used enterally after dilution.[66,104] Use immediately.[66] Follow the directions in section 3.6.

Trazodone

Presentation
Tablets, capsules.
Liquid.

Administration - enteral tubes / swallowing difficulties
1st choice – Use the liquid. Follow the directions in section 3.6.

Opening the capsules is not recommended but has been done.[84]
The contents of the capsules tastes unpleasant.[84] Follow the
directions in section 3.7. There is no information available about
crushing the tablets, so do not use.

Triapin

Presentation
Film-coated tablets.

Clinical guidance
Not suitable for administration via enteral feeding tubes. The
ingredients are light sensitive, and the formulation is modified-
release.[79] Contact Pharmacy for advice.

Trifluoperazine

Presentation
Coated tablets.
Solution (some preparations contain sorbitol).
Modified-release capsules.

Administration - enteral tubes / swallowing difficulties
Use the solution.[94,104,105] Follow the directions in section 3.6.

Trihexyphenidyl (Benzhexol)

Presentation
Tablets.
Syrup.

Administration - enteral tubes / swallowing difficulties
1st choice – Use the syrup.[41] Follow the directions in section 3.6.
2nd choice – The tablets have been crushed and mixed with water for administration.[133] Follow the directions in section 3.5.

Trimethoprim

Presentation
Tablets.
Suspension.
Injection.

Administration - enteral tubes / swallowing difficulties
1st choice – Give by parenteral injection if possible.
2nd choice – Use the suspension (contains sorbitol).[104] Follow the directions in section 3.6.

Feed guidance
Withhold enteral feeds for half an hour before and half an hour after each dose.[155]

Trimipramine

Presentation
Tablets, capsules.

Administration - enteral tubes / swallowing difficulties
The capsules can be opened and the contents dispersed in water for administration.[92] Follow the directions in section 3.7. Alternatively the tablets can be crushed.[92] Follow the directions in section 3.5. Both have a local anaesthetic action, so take care if used orally in patients with swallowing difficulties.[92]

Ursodeoxycholic acid

Presentation
Tablets, capsules.
Suspension.

Administration - enteral tubes / swallowing difficulties
1st choice – Use the suspension.[104] Follow the directions in section 3.6.
2nd choice – The tablets have been crushed and mixed with water for administration.[133] The powder resulting from crushing the tablets has limited solubility and may stick to the inside of enteral feeding tubes. If giving via enteral feeding tube, flush well after administration.[138] Follow the directions in section 3.5.

Valganciclovir

Presentation
Film-coated tablets.

Administration - enteral tubes
The tablets can be crushed and mixed with distilled water for administration. Crush well as the tablets are film-coated.[131] Follow the directions in section 3.5.

Administration - swallowing difficulties
The tablets can be crushed and mixed with distilled water or chocolate syrup for administration.[131] Follow the directions in section 3.5.

Valsartan

Presentation
Capsules.

Administration - enteral tubes / swallowing difficulties
The capsules can be opened, and the contents dispersed in water for administration.[85,104] Use immediately as the drug is not very stable.[104] If giving via enteral feeding tube, flush well after each dose as the capsule contents are not very soluble.[155] Follow the directions in section 3.7.

The capsule contents taste bitter.[85]

Vancomycin

Presentation
Capsules.
Injection.

Administration - enteral tubes / swallowing difficulties
1st choice – A solution can be made by Pharmacy. Follow the directions in section 3.6.
2nd choice – The injection can be diluted with 30ml water for injection and given enterally.[40,163] The expiry of the reconstituted injection depends upon the brand. Follow the directions in section 3.6.

Do not administer vancomycin capsules.

Clinical guidance
The indications for vancomycin injection and enteral vancomycin are different. Do not switch to the alternative route except on specialist advice. Contact Pharmacy for advice if necessary.

Venlafaxine

Presentation
Tablets.
Modified-release capsules.

Administration – enteral tubes
The tablets can be crushed and mixed with water for administration.[86] Follow the directions in section 3.5.

The modified-release capsules are not suitable for enteral tube administration.[86] Contact Pharmacy for advice on converting to standard tablets.

Administration – swallowing difficulties
Crushed tablets can be administered in jam for patients with swallowing difficulties.[105]

The modified-release capsules contain modified-release beads which can be emptied out and given in smooth food, e.g. yoghurt, for patients with swallowing difficulties. The beads must be swallowed whole, therefore this method may not be appropriate for patients with limited understanding / impaired ability to follow instructions.[105]

Verapamil

Presentation
Tablets.
Sugar-free oral solution.
Modified-release tablets, modified-release capsules.

Administration - enteral tubes / swallowing difficulties
1st choice – Use the oral solution. Follow the directions in section 3.6.
2nd choice – The standard tablets have been crushed and mixed with water for administration. They have a bitter taste and a local anaesthetic effect in the mouth.[105,152] Follow the directions in section 3.5.
3rd choice – The injection can be given enterally.[40,138,152] Follow the directions in section 3.6.

Do not crush the modified-release tablets or open the capsules.

Clinical guidance
Dose changes and frequency changes are required if changing from controlled release verapamil to the oral solution. Contact Pharmacy for advice.

Feed guidance
Give on an empty stomach, - withhold enteral feeds for one hour before and one hour after each dose.

Vigabatrin

Presentation
Film-coated tablets.
Sachets.

Administration - enteral tubes / swallowing difficulties
1st choice – Use the sachets.[104] Follow the directions in section 3.6.
2nd choice – The tablets can be crushed and dispersed in water for administration.[138,152] Follow the directions in section 3.5.

Vitamin B Co Strong

Presentation
Film-coated tablets.

Clinical guidance
Consider switching to Pabrinex injection or Vigranon B syrup (not available on NHS).[94,136] Contact Pharmacy for advice.

Vitamin E

Presentation
Suspension.

Administration - enteral tubes / swallowing difficulties
Use the suspension.[104] Follow the directions in section 3.6.

Voriconazole

Presentation
Film-coated tablets.
Oral suspension.
Intravenous infusion.

Administration - enteral tubes / swallowing difficulties
1st choice – Give by infusion if possible.
2nd choice – Use the suspension.[132] Follow the directions in section 3.6.
3rd choice – The tablets can be crushed and mixed with water for administration.[132] Follow the directions in section 3.5.

Warfarin

Presentation
Tablets.

Administration - enteral tubes / swallowing difficulties
1st choice – A suspension can be made by Pharmacy at some centres. Dilute the suspension with the same volume of distilled water before administration. Follow the directions in section 3.6.
2nd choice – The tablets can be crushed and mixed with water for administration.[38,41] Follow the directions in section 3.5.

Clinical guidance
Warfarin is available as a racemate of two enantiomers. One is much more potent than the other. As putting the tablets into solution will lead to an alteration in the proportions of the two enantiomers, care should be taken.[142] It is advisable to keep patients on a consistent formulation, and monitor the INR closely following any necessary changes. Warfarin has a low solubility at pH levels below 8, and precipitation may occur.[142]

Feed guidance
Withhold enteral feeds for one to two hours before and one to two hours after each dose.

Care is necessary when patients are also receiving enteral feeds with a high vitamin K content. Vitamin K in as little as 50mcg doses have been reported to antagonise the effects of warfarin, i.e. decrease prothrombin time,[33] though it generally requires a dose of 140-500mcg.[4]

Enteral feeds containing sufficient amounts of vitamin K for this interaction to occur include Ensure® (100mcg/ml),[34] Osmolite®, and Ensure Plus®.[11] The INR should be monitored closely and the warfarin dose adjusted as necessary.

Avoid feeds containing soya protein.[87]

Zaleplon

Presentation
Capsules.

Clinical guidance
Administration via enteral feeding tube is not recommended as the capsule contents are practically insoluble and would stain the tube.[138]

Zidovudine

Presentation
Capsules.
Film-coated tablets.
Syrup.
Injection.

Administration - enteral tubes / swallowing difficulties
Use the syrup.[41] Follow the directions in section 3.6.

Zinc sulphate

Presentation
Effervescent tablets.
Injection.

Administration - enteral tubes / swallowing difficulties
1st choice – Give by parenteral injection if appropriate.
2nd choice - Use the effervescent tablets.[94] Follow the directions in section 3.5.

Zolpidem

Presentation
Tablets.

Administration - enteral tubes / swallowing difficulties
The tablets can be crushed and mixed with water for administration.[104] Follow the directions in section 3.5.

Zopiclone

Presentation
Film-coated tablets.

Clinical guidance
The tablets are not suitable for crushing or dissolving, and should not be used, as the powder will thicken quickly and may block enteral feeding tubes. Contact Pharmacy for advice on alternatives.[62]

Zotepine

Presentation
Sugar coated tablets.

Clinical guidance
The tablets are small, sugar coated and difficult to crush. Administration via enteral feeding tube is not recommended.[138]

Zuclopenthixol

Presentation
Film-coated tablets.
Depot injections.

Administration - enteral tubes / swallowing difficulties
1st choice – A suspension may be made by Pharmacy at some centres.[138] Follow the directions in section 3.6.
2nd choice – The tablets can be crushed and mixed with water for administration.[104,105] They are film-coated and may block enteral feeding tubes. If giving via enteral feeding tube, flush well after administration. Follow the directions in section 3.5.

5. References

Please note that information obtained from pharmaceutical companies does not constitute a recommendation by that company that the drug is suitable for administration via an enteral feeding tube or to patients with swallowing difficulties. Such use is usually outside the drug licence, and most information is anecdotal.

1.   Chadwick C. Pharmaceutical problems for the nutrition team pharmacist. Hospital Pharmacist 1996; 3: 139-146.

2.   Varella. Drug Nutrients Interactions in Enteral Feeding: A primary care focus. The Nurse Practitioner 1997; 22: 98-104.

3.   Oxford Textbook of Medicine.pp1321. Third Edition. Edited by Weathcrall, DJ. Oxford University Press, 1996.

4.   Beckwith M. A guide to drug therapy in patients with enteral feeding tubes: Dosage form selection and administration methods. Hospital Pharmacy 1997; 32: 57-64.

5.   Cutie A. Compatibility of enteral products with commonly employed drug additives. Parental Enteral Nutrition 1983; 7: 186-191.

6.   Adams D. Administration of drugs through a jejunostomy tube. British Journal Intensive Care 1994; 4: 10-17.

7.   Mistry B. Simplifying oral drug therapy for patients with swallowing difficulties. Pharmaceutical Journal 1995; 254: 808-809.

8.   Martin T. Tablet dispersion as an alternative to formulation of oral liquid dosage form. Aust. J. Hospital Pharmacy 1993; 23: 378-386.

9.   Reynolds JEF, editor. Martindale: The Extra Pharmacoepia. 31st Edition London: Pharmaceutical Press, 1996.

10.   Clark-Schmidt A. Loss of carbamazepine suspension through nasogastric feeding tubes. Am.J.Hosp.Pharmacy 1990; 4: 2034-2037.

11.   Stockley IH. Drug Interactions. Fourth Edition. London: Pharmaceutical Press, 1996.

12. D'arcy P F. Drug interactions with medical plastics. ADR toxicol. review 1996; 15: 207-219.

13. Pharmacy Information Sheet. July 1997. Ciprofloxacin.

14. Hillcross: data on file (communication with Brenda Murphy).

15. Micromedex Healthcare Series, volume 104.

16. Lilly: Data on file (communication with Brenda Murphy).

17. Janssen: Data on file (communication with Brenda Murphy).

18. American Hospital Formulary Service. 1997.

19. Flagyl® Summary of Product Characteristics, 96/97. Hawgreen Ltd.

20. Liefold J. Administration of controlled–release morphine sulphate during artificial feeding. Z. Allg. Med. 1996; 76: 707-709.

21. Battino D et al. Clinical Pharmacokinetics of anti-epileptic drugs in paediatric patients. CPK 1995; 29: 341-369.

22. Dickerson R, Melnik G. Osmolality of oral solutions and suspensions. Am. J. Hosp. Pharm. 1998; 45: 832-834.

23. Miller SW, Strom JG. Stability of Phenytoin in three enteral nutrients formulas. Am. J. Hosp. Pharm. 1998; 45: 2529-2523.

24. Archer A. Guideline for nurses on drug administration through enteral feeding tubes Pharmacy Own Magazine 1996; 10: 2-3.

25. Holtz L. Compatibility of medications with enteral feeds. J. Par. Ent. Nutrition 1987; 11: 183-186.

26. Estoup M. Approaches and limitations of medication delivery in patients with enteral feeding tubes. Critical Care Nurse 1994; 14: 68-72.

27. Parke-Davis: Data on file (communication with Brenda Murphy).

28. Halpern NA. Segmental intestinal absorption of ranitidine: investigate and therapeutic implications. Am. J. Gastroenterology 1990; 85: 539-543.

29. Gramatte. Site dependent small intestinal absorption of ranitidine. Eur. J. Clin. Pharmacology 1994; 46: 253-259.

30. Zantac® Summary of Product Characteristics, 96/97. GlaxoWellcome UK.

31. Williams MF, et al. Influence of GI anatomic site of drug deliverance on the absorption characteristics of rantidine. Pharmacotherapy 1989; 9: 184.

32. Tomlin M, Dixon S. Aluminium and naosgastric feeds. (Letter) Pharmaceutical Journal 1995; 256: 40.

33. Mason P. Diet and drug interactions. Pharmaceutical Journal 1996; 255: 94-95.

34. Watson JM. Enteral feeds may antagonise warfarin. BMJ 1994; 288: 557.

35. BNF No. 42 (Sept. 2001). London: British Medical Association, Royal Pharmaceutical Society of Great Britain, 2001.

36. Ciproxin® Summary of Product Characteristics, 1999/2000. Bayer plc.

37. Personal communication, Medical information, Pfizer Limited, 10.8.01.

38. Nova laboratories Keltrol compatability bulletin.

39. Dispersal of non-soluble tabs in water (in-house work, Wrexham Maelor Hospital).

40. Tube Feeding Drug Administration Guide, Forest Healthcare, Whipps Cross Hospital, Leytonstone, London.

41. Derriford Hospital Pharmacy enteral feeding guide.

42. Personal communication, Medical Information, Sanofi-Synthelabo, 6.9.01.

43. Personal communication, Medical Information, Bayer, 16.8.01.

44. Personal communication, Medical Information, Boehringer Ingelheim, 14.8.01.

45. Personal communication, Medical Information, Servier, 6.9.01.

46. Personal communication, Medical Information, AstraZeneca, 14.8.01.

47. Printed information from Link Pharmaceuticals on Zomorph capsules.

48. Personal communication, Medical Information, Lilly, 16.8.01.

49. Personal communication, Medical Information, DuPont, 14.8.01.

50. Fosamax® Summary of Product Characteristics. MSD, Aug. 1997.

51. Arthrotec® Summary of Product Characteristics. Searle, June 1997.

52. Personal communication, Medical Information, Roche, 6.9.01.

53. Personal communication, Medical Information, AstraZeneca, 23.7.01.

54. Personal communication, Medical Information, Pharmacia, 6.9.01.

55. Personal communication, Medical Information, Pantheon, 16.8.01.

56. Personal communication, Medical Information, Abbott Laboratories, 13.8.01.

57. Personal communication, Medical Information, Pharmacia, 12.12.01.

58. Personal communication, Medical Information, AstraZeneca, 13.8.01.

59. Personal communication, Medical Informaton, Schering Health, 6.9.01.

60. Plendil® Summary of Product Characteristics. AstraZeneca, 1999/2000.

61. Personal communication, Medical Information, Fournier, 13.8.01.

62. Personal communication, Medical Information, Aventis Pharma, 14.8.01.

63. Personal communication, Medical Information, MSD, 6.9.01.

64. Proscar® Summary of Product Characteristics. MSD, Oct. 1998.

65. Personal communication, Medical Information, Novartis, 6.9.01.

66. Personal communication, Medical Information, Pharmacia, 19.9.01 (letter).

67. Personal communication, Medical Information, GlaxoSmithkline, 10.10.01.

68. Personal communication, Medical Information, Bristol-Myers Squibb, 14.8.01.

69. Personal communication, Medical Information, Napp, 13.8.01.

70. Tavanic® Summary of Product Characteristics. Aventis Pharma, Sept. 1998.

71. Personal communication, Medical Information, Pharmacia, 16.11.01.

72. Personal communication, Medical Information, Organon, 6.9.01.

73. Singulair® Summary of Product Characteristics. MSD, Jan. 1998.

74. Personal communication, Medical Information, Solvay Healthcare, 9.8.01.

75. Personal communication, Medical Information, Lilly, 16.8.01.

76. Coversyl® Summary of Product Characteristics. Servier, March 1997.

77. Personal communication, Medical Information, Bristol-Myers Squibb, 6.9.01.

78. Personal communication, Medical Information, Merck, 16.8.01, communication with Sioned Rowlands.

79. Personal communication, Medical Information, Aventis Pharma, 23.7.01.

80. Personal communication, Medical Information, Procter and Gamble Pharm., 16.8.01.

81. Personal communication, Medical Information, Smithkline Beecham, 3.8.01.

82. Flomax® Summary of Product Characteristics. Yamanouchi, July 1998.

83. Personal communication, Medical Information, Pharmacia, 10.10.01.

84. Personal communication, Medical Information, Aventis Pharma, 25.10.01.

85. Personal communication, Medical Information, Novartis, 29.6.01.

86. Personal communication, Medical Information, Wyeth, 6.9.01.

87. Engle K, Hannawa TE, Techniques for administering oral medications to critical care patients receiving continuous enteral nutrition. Am J Health-Syst Pharm. 1999; 56:1441-4.

88. Tenormin® Syrup Summary of Product Characteristics. Zeneca Pharma, February 1998.

89. Personal communication, Medical Information, Celltech, 10.10.01.

90. Thomson FC, Naysmith MR, Lindsay A. Managing drug therapy in patients receiving enteral and parenteral nutrition. Hospital Pharmacist 2000; 7:155-164.

91. Personal communication, Medical Information, Merck, 10.07.02.

92. Personal communication, Medical Information, Aventis Pharma, 11.07.02.

93. BNF No. 43 (March 2002). London: British Medical Association, Royal Pharmaceutical Society of Great Britain, 2002.

94. Queen Victoria Hospital's Drug Adminstration via Enteral Feeding Tubes guide, March 2001.

95. Thomson F. A to Z guide to administration of drugs via nasogastric/PEG tube. Southern General Hospital, Victoria Infirmary, South Glasgow University Hosptials NHS Trust, University of Strathclyde/GGHB Pharmacy Practice Unit, Western General Hospital, Lothian University Hospitals NHS Trust, University of Strathclyde/Lothian Pharmacy Practice Unit. June 2001.

96. Product Information, Catapres® Transdermal Plasters, Boehringer Ingelheim.

97. Personal communication, Medical Information, Borg Medicare, 27.9.02.

98. Personal communication, Medical Information, Waymed Healthcare, 27.9.02.

99. Personal communication, Medical Information, Celltech, 27.9.02.

100. Personal communication, Medical Information, Boehringer Ingelheim, 27.9.02.

101. Topamax Summary of Product Characteristics. Janssen-Cilag, 17.2.99.

102. Personal communication, Medical Information, Link Pharmaceuticals, 28.2.03.

103. Personal communication, Medical Information, Roche Consumer Health, 28.2.03.

104. Guidelines for the administration of Drugs through Enteral Feeding Tubes. County Durham and Darlington Acute Hospitals NHS Trust. 2nd edition. July 2003.

105. Drugs via Enteral Feeding Tubes Guide (draft copy), Stockport NHS Trust, received Sept. 2003.

106. BNF No. 45 (March 2003). London: British Medical Association, Royal Pharmaceutical Society of Great Britain, 2003.

107. Personal communication, Medical Information, Aventis Pharma, 24.12.03.

108. Personal communication, Medical Information, UCB Pharma, 12.2.04.

109. Personal communication, Medical Information, Goldshield, 15.1.04

110. Personal communication, Medical Information, Boehringer Ingelheim, 15.1.04.

111. Prograf® Summary of Product Characteristics. Fujisawa Ltd, June 2002.

112. Administering Drugs via Enteral Feeding Tubes: A Practical Guide. Poster produced by the British Association for Parenteral and Enteral Nutrition, and The British Pharmaceutical Nutrition Group, July 2004.

113. Drug Administration via Enteral Feeding Tubes: A Guide for General Practitioners and Community Pharmacists. Leaflet produced by the British Association for Parenteral and Enteral Nutrition, and The British Pharmaceutical Nutrition Group, July 2004.

114. Tube Feeding and Your Medicines: A Guide for Patients and Carers. Leaflet produced by the British Association for Parenteral and Enteral Nutrition, and The British Pharmaceutical Nutrition Group, July 2004.

115. Griffith R. Tablet Crushing and the Law. Pharmaceutical Journal 2003; 271: 90-91.

116. Wright D. Swallowing Difficulties Protocol: Achieving best practice in Medication Administration. 2002.

117. Carrington C, McKay J. Administering Drugs via Enteral Feeding Tubes. Pharmacy Department, Queensland, Australia. Nov. 2000.

118. MDA/2004/026 – Enteral feeding tubes (nasogastric). Safety alert produced by the Medicines and Healthcare products Regulatory Agency, 14th June 2004.

119. Anderson R. Personal correspondance, 10th May 2004.

120. Reducing the harm caused by misplaced nasogastric feeding tubes. National Patient Safety Agency, 21st February 2005.

121. Bird K. Is levothyroxine suspension effective? [letter] Pharmaceutical Journal 2004; 273: 680.

122. Perrin JH. Do not suspend levothyroxine. [letter] Pharmaceutical Journal 2004; 273: 748.

123. Cipramil® Summary of Product Characteristics. Lundbeck Limited, 25th Sept. 2003.

124. Personal communication, Medical Information, MSD. 8th June 2005.

125. Personal communication, Medical Information, Pfizer. 13th June 2005.

126. Personal communication, Medical Information, Roche. 16th Aug. 2005.

127. CellCept® Suspension Summary of Product Characteristics. Roche Products Limited, April 2005.

128. Personal communication, Medical Information, Leo Laboratories Limited. 16th Aug. 2005.

129. Rosemont Pharmaceuticals Specials List. July 2004.

130. Personal communication, Medical Information, Boehringer Ingelheim, 19th Aug. 2005.

131. Medical Information, Roche, via Katy Hand, St. Helier Hospital, Surrey, 26th Aug. 2005.

132. Guide to administration of medicines to patients with swallowing difficulties or feeding tubes (NG/PEG). Gloucestershire Hospitals NHS Foundation Trust. November 2004.

133. Sinden E. Drug Administration Guidelines. Poole Hospital NHS Trust Pharmacy Department, July 2002.

134. Communication from AstraZeneca Medical Information to Julie Davis, University Hospital of North Staffordshire NHS Trust, 3rd July 2003.

135. Martin S, Davidson R, Holland D. Medication and Enteral Feeding. Calderdale and Huddersfield NHS Trust, Febuary 2004.

136. BNF No. 49 (March 2005). London: British Medical Association, Royal Pharmaceutical Society of Great Britain, 2005.

137. Appendix 10. Palliativedrugs.com, 2002.

138. Reeves VJ. The Administration of medication via a Percutaneous Endoscopic Gastrostomy (PEG) tube. Pharmacy Department, Broomfield Hospital, Mid Essex Hospitals Services NHS Trust. March 2002.

139. Burnett L. Personal communication, 6th September 2005.

140. Working party for drug administration. Drug Administration via enteral tubes. University Hospital of North Staffordshire. Draft One, October 2003.

141. Temgesic® Summary of Product Characteristics. Schering-Plough Ltd, April 2004.

142. Information from Colin Ranshaw, Principal Pharmacist, Quality Assurance and Control, Cardiff.

143. Information from Mark Craig, Senior Clinical Pharmacist, Mayday University Hospital.

144. Information from Rachel Harries, Nevill Hall Hospital, Abergavenny, 4th February 2005.

145. Information from Christopher Livsey, Clinical Pharmacist, Royal Lancaster Infirmary.

146. Letter on file. Napp Pharmaceuticals.

147. Information on file, Wrexham Maelor Hospital Pharmacy Department.

148. Letter from Medical Information, AstraZeneca, 12th April 2000.

149. Communication with Elayne Harris, Area Pharmacy Specialist (Palliative Care), Glasgow, 4th February 2005.

150. Communication with Christopher Livsey, Clinical Pharmacist, Royal Lancaster Infirmary.

151. Communication with Jennifer Smith, Medicines Information Manager, North Staffordshire University Hospitals.

152. Medicines for Children, 2003. Royal College of Paediatrics and Child Health, Neonatal and Paediatric Pharmacists Group.

153. Losec MUPs® Patient Information Leaflet. AstraZeneca, March 2005.

154. In house data, July-August 2005.

155. Fair R, Proctor B. Administering Medicines Through Enteral Feeding Tubes. The Royal Hospitals, Belfast. 2nd edition.

156. Nexium® Summary of Product Characteristics. AstraZeneca UK Limited, October 2004.

157. Furazolidone Drug Evaluation. Micromedex Healthcare Series, Volume 126, 2005.

158. Adams D. Administration of drugs through a jejunostomy tube. British Journal of Intensive Care 1994: 10-17.

159. Personal communication, Medical Information, Roche, 11th October 2005.

160. BNF for children, 2005. London: BMJ Publishing Group Ltd, Royal Pharmaceutical Society of Great Britain, RCPCH Publications Ltd, 2005.

161. Personal communication, Medical Information, MSD, 25th November 2005.

162. Acitretin Safety Data Sheet. Roche, 02.09.03.

163. Vancocin CP Injection Summary of Product Characteristics. Flynn Pharma Ltd, 17th August 2001.

164. Personal communication, Medical Information, Link Pharmaceuticals, 4th January 2006.

165. Personal communication, Medical Information, Amdipharm, 4th January 2006.

166. Personal communication, Medical Information, Procter and Gamble, 4th January 2006.

167. Personal communication, Medical Information, Wockhardt UK, 4th January 2006.

168. Personal communication, Medical Information, 3M Healthcare, 4th January 2006.

169. Personal communication, Medical Information, Shire, 4th January 2006.

170. Personal communication, Medical Information, Boehringer Ingelheim, 4th January 2006.

171. Personal communication, Medical Information, GlaxoSmithkline, 4th January 2006.

172. Cyclophosphamide monograph. Lexi-Drugs. On-palm database, Lexi-Comp, 2005.

173. Procainamide monograph. Lexi-Drugs. On-palm databse, Lexi-Comp, 2005.
174. Metoprolol monograph. Lexi-Drugs. On-palm databse, Lexi-Comp, 2005.

175. Personal communication, Medical Information, AstraZeneca, 5th January 2006.

176. Theophyllines. McEvoy GK (editor). AHFS Drug Information, 2001. American Society of Health-System Pharmacists. Bethesda, MD, 2001.

6. Monograph index

Monograph index

Cefradine	64	Co-tenidone	86
Cefuroxime	65	Co-triamterzide	87
Celecoxib	65	Co-trimoxazole	87
Celiprolol	66	Cyclizine	88
Cetirizine	66	Cyclophosphamide	88
Chenodeoxycholic acid	66	Cyproterone	89
Chloral hydrate	67	Dantrolene	89
Chlorambucil	67	Dapsone	89
Chloramphenicol	67	Deflazacort	90
Chlordiazepoxide	68	Demeclocycline	90
Chloroquine	68	Desferrioxamine	90
Chlorothiazide	69	Desmopressin	91
Chlorphenamine	69	Dexamethasone	91
Chlorpromazine	70	Diazepam	92
Chlortalidone	70	Diazoxide	92
Ciclosporin	71	Diclofenac sodium	93
Cilazapril	71	Dicycloverine	93
Cimetidine	72	Didanosine	94
Cinnarizine	72	Digoxin	95
Ciprofibrate	73	Dihydrocodeine	96
Ciprofloxacin	74	Di-iodohydroxyquinoline	96
Citalopram	75	Diloxanide	96
Clarithromycin	75	Diltiazem	97
Clindamycin	76	Dinoprostone	97
Clobazam	76	Dipyridamole	98
Clomethiazole	77	Disodium etidronate	107
Clomipramine	77	Disopyramide	99
Clonazepam	78	Docusate	100
Clonidine	79	Domperidone	100
Clopidogrel	79	Donepezil	100
Clozapine	80	Dosulepin	101
Co-amilofruse	80	Doxazosin	101
Co-amilozide	80	Doxepin	102
Co-amoxiclav	81	Doxycycline	102
Co-beneldopa	82	Dydrogesterone	102
Co-careldopa	83	Efavirenz	103
Co-codamol	84	Emtricitabine	103
Co-danthramer	84	Enalapril	103
Codeine	84	Entacapone	104
Co-dydramol	84	Eprosartan	104
Co-fluampicil	85	Erythromycin	105
Colchicine	85	Escitalopram	105
Colestyramine	85	Esomeprazole	106
Combivir	86	Etamsylate	107
Co-phenotrope	86	Ethambutol	107

Ethosuximide	107	Hydroxyzine	126
Etoposide	108	Hyoscine butylbromide	126
Ezetimibe	108	Hyoscine hydrobromide	127
Famciclovir	108	Ibuprofen	127
Famotidine	109	Imipramine	128
Felodipine	109	Indapamide	128
Fenofibrate	109	Indometacin	129
Ferrous sulphate	109	Indoramin	129
Fexofenadine	110	Inositol nicotinate	130
Finasteride	110	Irbesartan	130
Flavoxate	110	Isoniazid	131
Flecainide	111	Isosorbide dinitrate	132
Flucloxacillin	112	Isosorbide mononitrate	133
Fluconazole	113	Isotretinoin	134
Fludrocortisone	113	Ispaghula husk	134
Fluoxetine	114	Isradipine	134
Flupentixol	114	Itraconazole	135
Fluphenazine	115	Ketoconazole	135
Flurbiprofen	115	Labetalol	136
Flutamide	115	Lacidipine	136
Fluvastatin	116	Lactulose	136
Fluvoxamine	116	Lamivudine	137
Folic acid	116	Lamotrigine	137
Forceval	117	Lansoprazole	138
Fosinopril	117	Leflunomide	139
Furazolidone	117	Lercanidipine	139
Furosemide	118	Levetiracetam	140
Gabapentin	118	Levofloxacin	140
Galantamine	119	Levomepromazine	141
Ganciclovir	119	Levothyroxine	142
Glibenclamide	120	Linezolid	143
Gliclazide	120	Lisinopril	143
Glimepiride	121	Lisuride	144
Glipizide	121	Lithium	144
Gliquidone	121	Lofepramine	145
Glyceryl trinitrate	122	Loperamide	145
Glycopyrronium	123	Loratadine	145
Granisetron	123	Lorazepam	146
Haloperidol	124	Lormetazepam	146
Hydralazine	124	Losartan	146
Hydrocortisone	125	Magnesium glycerophosphate	147
Hydromorphone	125	Mebendazole	147
Hydroxycarbamide	125	Mebeverine	147
Hydroxychloroquine	126	Medroxyprogesterone	148

Mefenamic acid	148	Neomycin	169
Mefloquine	148	Neostigmine	169
Megestrol acetate	149	Nicardipine	169
Melatonin	149	Niclosamide	170
Meloxicam	150	Nicorandil	170
Menadiol	150	Nifedipine	170
Meprobamate	150	Nimodipine	172
Meptazinol	151	Nitrazepam	172
Mercaptamine	151	Nitrofurantoin	173
Mercaptopurine	151	Nizatidine	173
Mesalazine	152	Norethisterone	173
Metformin	153	Norfloxacin	174
Methionine	153	Ofloxacin	174
Methotrexate	154	Olanzapine	175
Methylcellulose	154	Olsalazine	175
Methyldopa	155	Omeprazole	176
Methylphenidate	155	Ondansetron	177
Methylprednisolone	156	Orlistat	177
Metoclopramide	156	Orphenadrine	178
Metolazone	156	Oxcarbazepine	178
Metoprolol	157	Oxprenolol	178
Metronidazole	158	Oxybutynin	179
Metyrapone	159	Oxycodone	179
Mexiletine	159	Oxytetracycline	180
Mianserin	159	Pancreatin	181
Midazolam	160	Pantoprazole	181
Midodrine	160	Paracetamol	182
Minocycline	160	Paroxetine	182
Minoxidil	161	Penicillamine	183
Mirtazepine	161	Pentazocine	183
Misoprostol	162	Pentoxyfylline	184
Moclobemide	162	Peppermint Oil	184
Montelukast	163	Pergolide	184
Morphine	163	Pericyazine	185
Moxisylate	164	Perindopril	185
Moxonidine	165	Perphenazine	185
Multivitamins	165	Pethidine	186
Mycophenolate mofetil	166	Phenelzine	186
Nabilone	166	Phenobarbital	186
Nabumetone	167	Phenyoxybenzamine	187
Nadolol	167	Phenoxymethylpenicllin	183
Naftidrofuryl oxalate	167	Phenytoin	188
Nalidixic acid	168	Phosphate	190
Naproxen	168	Phytomenadione	190
Nefopam	168	Pimozide	190

Pioglitazone	191	Ropinerole	209
Piracetam	191	Rosiglitazone	209
Piroxicam	191	Rosuvastatin	209
Pizotifen	192	Salbutamol	210
Potassium chloride	192	Saquinavir	210
Pramipexole	193	Secobarbital	211
Pravastatin	193	Selegiline	211
Prazosin	193	Senna	211
Prednisolone	194	Sertraline	212
Pregabalin	194	Sildenafil	212
Primaquine	194	Simeticone	212
Primidone	195	Simvastatin	213
Probenecid	195	Sodium bicarbonate	213
Procainamide	195	Sodium chloride	213
Procarbazine	196	Sodium clodronate	214
Prochlorperazine	196	Sodium cromoglicate	214
Procyclidine	197	Sodium fusidate	215
Proguanil	197	Sodium phenylbutyrate	215
Promazine	197	Sodium picosulfate	215
Promethazine hydrochloride	198	Sodium valproate	216
Propafenone	198	Sotalol	216
Propantheline	198	Spironolactone	217
Propranolol	199	Stanozolol	217
Propylthiouracil	199	Stavudine	217
Pseudoephedrine	200	Sucralfate	218
Pyrazinamide	200	Sulfasalazine	219
Pyridostigmine	201	Sulindac	219
Pyridoxine	201	Sulpiride	219
Pyrimethamine	201	Tacrolimus	220
Quetiapine	202	Tamoxifen	220
Quinidine	202	Tamsulosin	221
Quinine sulphate	203	Telmisartan	221
Rabeprazole	203	Temazepam	222
Raloxifene	203	Tenofovir	222
Ramipril	204	Terazosin	222
Ranitidine	205	Terbinafine	223
Reboxetine	205	Tetrabenazine	223
Repaglinide	206	Tetrahydrobiopterin	223
Rifampicin	206	Thalidomide	224
Riluzole	207	Theophylline	224
Risedronate	207	Thiamine	225
Risperidone	207	Thioridazine	226
Ritonavir	208	Tiabendazole	226
Rivastigmine	208	Tiagabine	226

Tinidazole	227		
Tioguanine	227		
Tizanidine	227		
Tolbutamide	228		
Tolterodine	228		
Topiramate	229		
Torasemide	229		
Tramadol	230		
Trandolapril	230		
Tranexamic acid	230		
Trazodone	231		
Triapin	231		
Trifluoperazine	231		
Trihexyphenidyl	232		
Trimethoprim	232		
Trimipramine	232		
Ursodeoxycholic acid	233		
Valganciclovir	233		
Valsartan	234		
Vancomycin	234		
Venlafaxine	235		
Verapamil	236		
Vigabatrin	236		
Vitamin B Co Strong	237		
Vitamin E	237		
Voriconazole	237		
Warfarin	238		
Zaleplon	239		
Zidovudine	239		
Zinc sulphate	239		
Zolpidem	240		
Zopiclone	240		
Zotepine	240		
Zuclopenthixol	241		